CHEERS TO CHILDBIRTH

A DAD'S GUIDE TO CHILDBIRTH SUPPORT

LUCY PERRY

PURE PUBLISHING

For Hudson for making me into a mother in the first place,
Harlow for giving me the best birth story ever and
Sheba for adding just the right amount of chaos to our household.

First published 2010
Copyright Lucy Perry, 2010

Published by Pure Publishing
PO Box 5066 Turramurra NSW 2074
emailus@purepublishing.com.au

www.cheerstochildbirth.com.au

Cover image by Kate Buchner, Uber Photography
Photography in content provided by subject except where stated
Cover and text design by Adam Dipper, Pure Graphics Pty Limited

Printed in Australia by Griffin Press

National Library of Australia Cataloguing-in-Publication data:
Perry, Lucy
ISBN 978-0-9804132-1-2
Author: Perry, Lucy.
Title: Cheers to childbirth: a dad's guide to childbirth support
by Lucy Perry

ISBN: 9780980413212 (pbk.)

Subjects: Childbirth – Anecdotes.
            Fathers.
Dewey Number: 618.4

CONTENTS

Foreword by Dr Ric Porter   xi

Preface   xv

Introduction   1

PART ONE

Chapter 1: The expectant father's job description   9

Our birth stories   19

Chapter 2: Call for reinforcements   29

Paul Treseder's story   39

Chapter 3: What to say and what not to say during childbirth 43

Paul Osborne's story   55

Chapter 4: Understanding labour pain   59

James Tomkins' story   71

Chapter 5: Practical ideas for pain management   77

Danny Green's story   91

Chapter 6: Supporting your partner through loss   95

David Galilee's story   103

Chapter 7: How to be an advocate for your family   111

Digby Hone's story   119

PART TWO

Chapter 8: Prelabour   127

    Adam Spencer's story   137

Chapter 9: First stage of labour   143

    Charlie Teo's story   153

Chapter 10: Transition – duck for cover!   159

    Mark Occhilupo's story   165

Chapter 11: The big push and the moment of birth   169

    Mark Ferguson's story   179

Chapter 12: Third stage of labour   183

    Tim Vincent's story   189

Chapter 13: After the birth: the first few hours   195

    Jud Arthur's story   203

Chapter 14: Caesareans   207

    Gerrard Gosens' story   215

PART THREE

Chapter 15: Life after birth   221

    David Maxwell's story   235

Chapter 16: Breastfeeding for blokes   241

    Mike Baird's story   249

Afterword   255

Resources   256

Recommended reading   259

Acknowledgements   261

Notes   263

Bibliography   265

Index   266

FOREWORD

It is often said that a man can never say or do the right thing for his partner in labour. Perhaps this is because there has never been a significant resource to equip a man for one of the biggest days of his life. Lucy Perry is set to rectify the situation with this book.

My experience as a birthing father is little different from most. As a young registrar in training to be a specialist obstetrician, I thought I knew most of the science of labour and childbirth, but when my wife Amanda's waters broke at 5.30am, three days before her due date, I could not get her to hospital fast enough to the care of the midwives with whom I had trained. The next eight hours were full on, with regular strong contractions. Although I knew what was happening physiologically, I found it difficult to find the right words of emotional support. One midwife uttered a memorable line to Amanda: 'Well, you know what's going on, you're an obstetrician's wife!' Amanda is a lawyer: nothing was further from the truth for her. I had to change from obstetrician to carer and protector – and quickly!

By 5.30pm it was clear that my nearly 4kg daughter was too big for my 151cm tall wife. Amanda's cervix had only minimally dilated, the baby's head was still unengaged despite strong, regular contractions and there were signs of foetal distress. It was time for the bypass option – a Caesarean. The delivery was somewhat surreal as two of my good friends were performing the surgery. Our daughter Katie was lifted gently out and I was blown away; she was pink and noisy and gorgeous. My wife and I were both in tears.

Baby number two was easy for me. I was overseas! Amanda went into labour at 37 weeks, two weeks ahead of her planned repeat Caesar, by which time I had expected to be back home. The anaesthetist and nursing colleagues acted as surrogate husband and support crew and I met my son Hugh a few days later at the airport. I still haven't lived that one down.

The third and final baby was a doddle. A repeat Caesar that was expected, planned, organised and stress free. I know many would disapprove and say how unnatural and interventionist, but for Amanda and me the destination was far more important than the journey. The birth day was a buzz, an almost party-like atmosphere in the operating theatre and we agreed we had completed our family on a high with another gorgeous daughter, Polly.

In my professional experience of over 30 years and 5,000 deliveries, I think I have run the entire gamut of expectant fathers' personalities, reactions and responses to their partner's labour. Some fathers-to-be just do not want to be present and in fact become negative influences on the whole birthing experience. Some fathers have done their homework and planned extensively for the day. They become an integral part of the event and are a true asset to their partner. The majority fall between these groups, keen to be supportive but not having a clue where to begin their preparation. The certainty is that becoming a father changes your life and it makes sense to consider how you want that change to feel.

The personal accounts that Lucy has gathered in this book are true blokey insights into labour, birth and couple relationships. I think there is no doubt that a well prepared and supportive dad is worth his weight in pethidine! Men can possess the skills to make the whole 'ordeal' of labour the positive experience most couples hope for. Obstetricians and midwives would do well to include dads in all aspects of birthing: explanation, discussion and joint decision-making. Our role should be adjunctive and not directional.

I would be lying if I said I agreed with all that has been written about labour and birth in this book, but that's because there remain many subjective elements about the entire event. Birth is not all about evidence-based medicine. In my experience the couples who speak in the most positive terms about their experience are those who were flexible in their birth plan. They researched, they discussed, they knew all the options available to them and were prepared to experiment in labour with what worked for them. It's very hard to be dogmatic about a plan when you haven't even experienced your first painful contraction!

So many times men feel ill equipped to help their partner in their time of need. They crave the stories of their mates' experiences but are often too 'male' to ask. It is refreshing to read real case histories from role models such as Paul, Adam, Mark and the others. These are men accomplished in their own field but each story shows that childbirth is a very levelling, humbling and hugely personal experience. It does not just come naturally. These accounts not only provide an honest insight into labour from a man's perspective but are a real resource for future dads. No husband has ever said to me that he knew too much before the event!

I like to remind my patients that childbirth lasts hours and parenting lasts a lifetime. With Lucy Perry's contribution to preparing dads for these emotional hours I believe she will be starting them on the right path to the bigger issues of co-parenting healthy, happy children.

Dr Ric Porter
Obstetrician and fertility specialist

PREFACE

Since 2004, my husband Bruce and I have run Beer + Bubs: childbirth education sessions for men at the pub, hence the title of this book.

As a venue, the pub provides men with a familiar environment (their natural habitat some might say) in which to learn something very new and unfamiliar. It provides a casual atmosphere where expectant fathers are willing to ask the questions they may have hesitated to ask in hospital antenatal classes and where they can build a sense of camaraderie with other men in the same father-to-be boat. Beer + Bubs began in Sydney and are now held in pubs all over Australia.

After one of our first workshops, one of the men came up to me and said, 'Where's the book?' He hadn't expected to learn so much, hadn't thought to take notes and knew he'd have little chance of remembering it all when it came to the crunch. So it was his question that inspired me to write this book.

To each workshop we invite a father who has been to a previous Beer + Bubs session to come to the pub and tell his story. Some of the most common feedback we receive is that men really like hearing stories from other men who describe the experience as it was for them. This led me to include birth stories from fifteen Australian fathers from diverse backgrounds and made writing the book quite an adventure!

If you like the idea of heading to the pub in the name of childbirth, visit www.beerandbubs.com.au for details.

INTRODUCTION

The day that your child is born is one day in the life of your family that *you really can't afford to stuff up.*

When your partner is pregnant, you're at the beginning of one of life's most challenging but rewarding roller coaster rides: from the early, nauseous days of pregnancy (not to mention the challenges of IVF, if that was your journey) and watching your partner's belly grow as her emotional state becomes more fragile, through to facing the challenges of childbirth together, and then a lifetime of parenting. While parenting can be taken one day at a time, calling on expert advice when you need it and with room to practise, the day that your partner gives birth for the first time has no dress rehearsal.

This book is written to help expectant dads move childbirth from being a spectator sport to an event in their lives where they are as important to their partner as any medical team; where they go on a challenging journey as a couple that will enrich their relationship in powerful ways. The birth can be an experience where a father begins to bond with his child from the very first breath, a bond that will last forever. And it's a day in a man's life when it's completely OK to cry.

Cheers to Childbirth is relevant to couples whether they birth at home or in a hospital. About 99% of births in Australia take place in hospitals, so this is the environment referred to throughout the text. However, my recommendations for how best to support your partner are still relevant for homebirth dads. I've had two homebirths myself.

Unlike their fathers, men in the twenty-first century are welcome to be present at the births of their babies. The only problem is that no one has told them what to do in order to help and not to hinder the process.

Women can be complicated creatures at the best of times, so throw in a cocktail of unfamiliar hormones, a mountain of pain and a prize at the end that has more emotional investment than anyone ever imagined, and men have a huge challenge on their hands.

In the past, childbirth was secret women's business. In pre-modern times, the chicks would rally around when a woman went into labour, offering their support and knowledge to help her birth her baby, while the lads waited elsewhere for the good news. The advent of modern obstetrics booted this ancient, experienced, female support from the birthing mother's circle and replaced it with male-led medical management. This still kept fathers out of the picture. We have a lot to thank modern obstetrics for, but fathers were excluded from childbirth for far too long.

In the 1970s, fathers were invited into the labour ward to witness the birth of their baby and support their partner through childbirth. I was born in the early '70s and my father witnessed my birth. I was the youngest of four and mine was the only birth he was allowed to be present at: the nuns shooed him away when he dropped my mother off at the hospital for the births of my older siblings. 'It's a girl!' he hollered when he laid eyes on me. According to my mum, this was the only contribution he was able to make.

In the twenty-first century, attitudes have changed in a big way. In fact, there is now a social expectation that men attend the birth of their babies. What used to be the secret business of the women's circle is now the expectant father's job description.

French surgeon Dr Michel Odent suggests that men shouldn't be involved in childbirth[1], because they 'make busy' in the moments after the birth when a woman should just be gazing into the eyes of her baby, producing the natural hormones that promote breastfeeding. He also suggests that men are not emotionally equipped to cope with such an event as the birth of their offspring and that they talk too much[2].

Dr Odent also believes that men can't help being anxious when their partner is in labour and that this fear rubs off on their partner, hampering her progress and making the birth more painful.

We'll forgive Dr Odent for declaring that fathers have no place at birth as he has written some landmark books and is widely regarded as a champion of mother-centred care, introducing birthing pools into French maternity hospitals in the 1970s and '80s. He's a man ahead of his time.

What *is* detrimental to a woman's progress in labour and bonding with her newborn is a bloke who has no clue: a dad who's madly texting his sisters for advice, taking photos 'down the business end', asking the obstetrician what the footy scores are or just ducking for cover when the going gets tough, rather than massaging his partner's aching back for hours and hours and knowing when to zip it. If those are the men that Dr Odent would like to keep out of labour wards all over the world, he's absolutely right.

It is true that men who talk too much during their partner's labour distract her from the task at hand. If a man can't control his own anxiety and fear, this does have a physical impact on a labouring woman and her hormones, working to slow down the progress of her labour and hamper her natural pain management chemistry.

According to Associate Professor of Midwifery, Hannah Dahlen of the University of Western Sydney, most men are a great asset to their partner in labour. 'A woman's partner is the person that she feels most comfortable with. He's someone that she has shared many experiences with and is a man that she trusts,' says Hannah.

'However, a small number of men – perhaps more than we know because men don't like to talk about it – are terrified of being present at the birth of their baby and desperately don't want to be there. If a man is forced to be with his partner in labour, his fear can impact on the woman's experience and can effectively alter the course of the birth in a negative way.'

If this sounds like you and you would rather have root canal therapy than be at the birth, if those fears are genuine and will prevent you from being totally emotionally available to your partner, you need to have a long think about whether your presence will have a positive impact on the birth and provide a good start to your role as a father. If, in all honesty, you recognise that your presence would probably not be helpful, you will need to find a person whom you both trust, preferably an experienced birth attendant, to support your partner.

'We need a get-out clause for men,' says Hannah. 'They shouldn't be forced to be involved in childbirth if they don't want to be. Most men are keen to be involved, but men are doers and women are talkers, thinkers and feelers. Birth is an incredibly instinctive process and men need to allow this process to unfold without trying to fix anything.'

You may be undecided about the expectant father's job description and what your role might be. This book will clear that up for you.

By supporting your partner in the right ways (and as you will see, some of these ways are not what the average man would expect) you can harness your partner's natural hormone production so that labour progresses smoothly and her pain is managed by floods of magic endorphins. Behave badly in the birth suite and your partner's body will produce adrenalin, the hormone that blocks the good hormones designed to drive the labour and manage the pain. In a nutshell, if you are a bozo at the birth, you will make the labour longer and harder for your partner.

So, what are my qualifications for writing this book? Firstly, I've given birth to three babies of my own so I know how it feels to push something that weighs four kilograms through the birth canal. Those experiences have given me first hand knowledge so that I can explain to you what your partner is going through, how it feels and how you can help. I've had a hospital birth and two homebirths.

I am also a certified doula or birth attendant. Labour coach if you will. I've attended many births as a doula and seen birth unfold in many different ways. I've supported women who have had natural vaginal births, medicated births, Caesareans, water births, super fast births, slow births, forceps deliveries, vacuum extractions, effortless births and labours that are long and hard. I doubt I have seen it all, with the huge variation of birth experiences being the only common element among all the couples I have supported.

It was in this role that I noticed that men are so often left out when it comes to preparing for the birth of their child. They want to be involved, but they don't necessarily know how to do this effectively.

I'm not a midwife and this book is not aiming to prepare you for a role in midwifery. This book is really Doula 101 for Dads. You won't be taking your partner's blood pressure or noting down the baby's heart beat during the birth; instead you'll be massaging her back, giving her sips of water and saying all the right things to reassure her. That's a special role you'll be fulfilling.

I'm also married to a man and fifteen years of marriage has taught me that men are *really bad mind readers*. They much prefer you to tell it to them straight and give them practical, useful information. When it comes to childbirth, men don't want to hear 'imagine you are your foetus, travelling down the birth canal' metaphors. They just want to know what they need to do in order to have a positive role in the births of their babies. That's what I'm best at – telling it to you straight, without the fluff.

This book has been written to spell out exactly what is expected of you at the birth of your baby and how you can make it an easier experience for the birthing mother, while making it a rewarding and memorable experience for you both.

Each chapter ends with a summary and is followed by a unique birth story from a man who has been through the gates of fatherhood before.

Most of these men are well known Australians who are highly successful in their field. Their fascinating, hilarious and sometimes heart breaking stories show that no matter how successful a man is, he faces the same challenges as any other guy when his partner gives birth.

Cheers to Childbirth should be read in addition to attending an antenatal course in childbirth. Hopefully, you'll find these classes fascinating. On the other hand, you may be bored to snores by six or seven weeks of content that is all about your partner's obstetric ins and outs, but she will love you for it and that's a good start. Though having you there is important for your partner, expectant fathers don't need volumes of technical detail. For this reason, in this book the obstetric explanations of the birth process are brief. You won't find cross-sectional diagrams of the female anatomy in the pages to come.

I recommend that, as well as reading this book and attending an antenatal course, expectant dads prepare for childbirth by watching as many birth videos as they can lay their hands on. Some cable channels have time slots dedicated to birth videos ranging from fascinating to downright gory. I think it is important that you see a baby emerging from the body of a woman on film before you see this happening to your partner. Once you've seen this happen 10 or 20 times, it's not that big a deal. Rather than being shocked by what you see, you'll be able to enjoy the fascinating emergence of a new life: your own child.

You're on quite a learning curve. Just remember that you have the power to make the birth process easier for your beloved with the words you use and the way you touch her during labour. So read on, discover what other men have discovered before you and prepare for what could be one of the most miraculous days of your life.

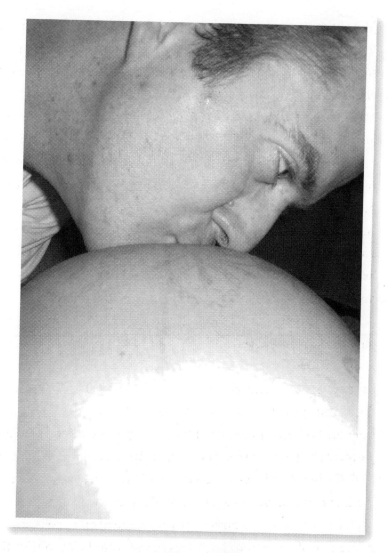

PART ONE

CHAPTER ONE

THE EXPECTANT FATHER'S JOB DESCRIPTION

Having this book in your hand suggests that you want to be more than a helpless onlooker at your baby's birth. That's an excellent start because being involved in a hands-on, positive way will bring immediate and ongoing rewards to your partner, your child and yourself. Your involved presence has the potential to enhance the relationship you have with your partner. You think you love her now? Wait until she delivers your baby. You'll love her in a whole new way that includes admiration, a new kind of respect and an enormous amount of gratitude for what she has done for you and what she's been through in the process.

You'll also have a better foundation for bonding with your baby if you're an active member of the birthing team. Your baby already knows the sound of your voice, so your comfort will be the next best thing after the child's mother in those first moments after your baby enters the world. Make the most of the opportunity to start your role as a father in a hands-on, loving and emotional way by being as involved as possible in the entire birth process.

Being a childbirth support person is like being on the support crew for a marathon runner: it's long and tiring and you have to put in planning and preparation. You need to stay positive and encouraging, even when you wish you could take a nap, changing your support to suit the stage of the race. You're in this together but when it comes to the crunch, she's the one who has to push across the finish line. Childbirth, however, is not a race and your partner can't back out when the going gets tough.

Dealing with other people's opinions

The job of the support crew starts many months before the event and for many expectant fathers, the job begins with fielding judgemental comments from others. You may have noticed during your partner's pregnancy that childbirth can be a touchy subject. Announce at a backyard barbecue that you and your partner are planning an all-natural water birth with no epidural and watch how fast those who have had an epidural slam your plans as ludicrous. 'Take the drugs! Take the drugs!' a complete stranger said to me once when I was almost nine months pregnant and waddling into a restaurant. 'You're very brave,' others said when we had decided on a homebirth for our second and third babies. On the other hand, just wait for the all-natural earth mothers to gasp if you say you're opting for a medically managed birth with an early epidural!

For a very personal and private event in your life, your preferences are nobody's business but yours as a couple, but the choices surrounding childbirth seem to draw opinions from every direction. Even newspaper columnists like to rant about what they think is the selfishness of couples who prefer to birth at home or, at the other end of the scale, branding women who choose a Caesarean as 'too posh to push'.

The reality is that others feel validated if you make the same choices as they did. But it's not your job to make others feel better about their childbirth choices. Your job as support partner (and that role started as soon as your partner became pregnant) is to ignore judgement, make choices together as a couple to provide the healthiest possible passage into the world for your child and reinforce your partner's confidence in her ability to birth. This means you have to become skilled at changing the subject, filing all judgemental comments in the 'thanks for coming' box while as a couple you stay focused on your preferences for the birth.

Childbirth horror stories are another destructive social force that you need to fend off in the lead-up to the birth. It seems that a pregnant belly comes with a neon sign that says, 'Tell me your childbirth horror stories!' or even worse, 'Haven't dealt with your childbirth baggage? Offload it on me!' A woman needs absolute confidence in herself and her body to give birth effectively, so frightening her with gory and exaggerated birth stories will only hamper her ability to prepare to give birth with trust and self-assuredness.

Some women who have had traumatic births find it helpful to retell their story in order to process their trauma, but you and your pregnant partner need to focus on preparing for your birth rather than helping others to work through their own negative experiences. Women birthing for the first time need to be aware that childbirth is hard work and it's not all aromatherapy and candles, but allowing your partner to be frightened by horror stories is counterproductive.

Sure, childbirth is tough, even traumatic for some, but for most women it's no horror story. Some women *love* giving birth. Some even have orgasms during childbirth!

Writing a birth plan

You may wish to write a birth plan together with your partner in the months before the birth. The process of writing a birth plan will give you both a chance to discuss your preferences and come to an agreement on the choices you have available to you when your partner gives birth. It's important to make sure that a birth plan doesn't set you up for unrealistic expectations and that it remains flexible.

Sydney obstetrician, Dr John Keogh, says that he is concerned when he sees a couple with a very detailed and rigid birth plan: 'If I'm handed a twenty-page volume for a birth plan with flowers and butterflies drawn in the margins, I get worried. Rigid plans have a way of getting in the way in childbirth. I tell my patients to keep their preferences in mind and to make them known but to go into the birth with an open mind. To go with the flow. It's like parenting, really. You think your son will be a footballer like you but all he wants to do is dance. You've got to change your plan. Some women feel like a failure if they don't achieve their ideal birth but this can be avoided if couples approach the birth with a flexible plan.'

Dr Keogh's flexible plan is a good idea. As you will see in the birth stories told in the pages of this book – just about anything can happen. Childbirth is a wonderful, miraculous event but there are so many variables that can happen on the journey to birth and a birth plan can't cover every variable.

I met a couple once who interviewed me with a view to engaging me as their doula. They were using project management software to manage their birth, with separate schedules for preparing the nursery, managing doctor's appointments and, believe it or not, a schedule for labour! She was a website developer and he was a construction project manager. They honestly thought that they could manage the flow of labour on their laptops.

I warned them that labour isn't something to which you could allocate little coloured squares in a spreadsheet, that it is an organic, natural event that can be unpredictable. They stopped typing and looked up from their laptops. They had been interviewing me against a set of key performance indicators as if I were going for a top job. According to their birth plan, they wanted a natural birth with no medical intervention and a short labour. 'And we're very organised people,' she confirmed. I could see that! However, they were completely unrealistic in their expectations of childbirth and were setting themselves up for disappointment. There were no surprises when I didn't get the gig to support them.

If you write a birth plan, keep it to a one-page summary of your childbirth preferences and give this to your caregivers who will include it in your notes, which are supposed to be referenced when your partner is in labour. Birth consultant Denise Love believes that a birth plan should be written just for yourselves, to help you discuss all your options and make choices in terms of your birth wishes: 'Midwives and obstetricians have enough on their plates already without reading volumes of birth wishes as well. Keep your birth plan short and sweet and use it as a tool to help you and your partner discuss your wishes for the birth so that you both know where you stand.' The last thing you want during the labour is to discover that you and your partner disagree on something such as the drugs you're willing or not willing to opt for.

You may also wish to talk about and include in your birth plan how your partner feels about her modesty. She needs to approach the birth with absolute confidence, but many women struggle with the reality that their modesty may feel shot to pieces during the process. If protecting her modesty is important to your partner, you can assure her that there is no reason why she can't be relatively decent while she's in labour. This is a very real and valid fear for some women who are not comfortable with baring all to people they don't know.

I once had a woman ask me whether she could keep her undies on for the birth. She was a deeply religious woman and the thought of being naked in a room with medical professionals in attendance was terrifying for her. Your partner will need to reveal everything from the waist down once she is pushing out the baby but she can keep a T shirt or hospital gown on right through the birth. There's no reason why she has to be starkers unless she's completely comfortable with that.

There are various online birth plans available or you can ask for a birth plan outline from the childbirth educator who presents your antenatal classes. Your caregivers may not have the time to review your birth plan before you arrive at the hospital with your labouring partner so just remind the midwife of your general birth wishes when you meet.

Your relationship with your partner's caregivers
In the lead up to the birth you and your partner will develop a

relationship with your caregivers. This may be an obstetrician who will deliver your baby in a private hospital, a team of midwives in a public hospital or an independent midwife who'll assist you to birth at home.

Here's the truth about your caregivers.

Your partner's obstetrician is a highly trained, specialised medical practitioner whose overriding goal is to make sure your baby survives the journey through the birth canal and that your partner is well and able to have babies again in the future. Obstetricians want healthy outcomes before they want champagne and roses. Their work is very demanding and they may well have to run from operating on a woman with a life-threatening ectopic pregnancy to an emergency Caesarean and then on to a totally straightforward vaginal birth, without skipping a beat. So don't rely on them to give you warm, fuzzy feelings about the birth of your baby. They're also, understandably, more interested in the pregnant woman in this relationship than in the baby's father, so don't be surprised if you feel a little on the outer.

I had an expectant dad in one of my workshops who was distressed that he had been to see the obstetrician with his partner for several prenatal visits, taking the time off work to accompany her each time, and yet the obstetrician hadn't given him eye contact or even a handshake. While it would be more pleasant to be acknowledged, approach your relationship with the obstetrician without having expectations that he or she will necessarily include you in that relationship. You're the man who pays the bill: don't expect a cuddle.

Sydney obstetrician, Dr Gary Sykes, encourages fathers to be involved throughout the process from antenatal visits right through to the moment of birth. 'I like meeting the father-to-be and take interest in his career and other aspects of his life. I think it's important that we meet and that we have a good rapport,' says Gary. 'I've always felt that a good relationship between an obstetrician and the father is essential to caring well for a woman.'

If your partner's obstetrician is blessed with a fabulous manner and an inclusive attitude, as well as the smarts to do what he or she does for a living, then you are more likely to be included in the process and given a hands-on role.

As Dr John Keogh says, 'The baby's father, the midwives and the obstetrician make up an important team that has to work together with the pregnant woman at its centre. As long as the woman is at the centre of what we are all doing to support her, she will feel safe and protected and can give birth with confidence.'

Obstetricians have copped some criticism in the past for being insensitive, for bullying women into interventions they didn't want and for ignoring fathers. According to Dr Gary Sykes, this behaviour is predominantly a thing of the past but some obstetricians still treat their patients with a lack of inclusion in the process. 'In the past, attitudes were very different from what they are today. Doctors were usually not questioned and could make very important decisions without consideration of the woman and her preferences. There was minimal discussion and a more dictatorial attitude in those days,' says Gary. 'Doctors such as these would find it very hard to survive in today's world. This is true not just in obstetrics but in medicine in general.'

Dr Sykes is a father of three himself and switched from pediatrics to obstetrics for the love of babies and the magical process of birth and concedes that his patients and their partners require special care. 'Men and women think very differently and for a male doctor to see things from the woman's perspective takes listening, sensitivity and time.'

Many men reading this book will be supporting their partner to give birth in a public hospital with a team of midwives caring for her. Midwives are often working understaffed, particularly in the public system, and can be running from one birth suite to the next, delivering babies one after the other, then following up with a mountain of paperwork. There's often little or no time for midwives to give couples the emotional support they need and unprepared or anxious fathers can sometimes be seen as a hindrance to getting the job done properly. If your timing is good and the birth unit is not too busy, the midwife will be able to spend more time with you and your partner.

One-on-one care with a midwife within the public hospital system or birthing at home with an independent midwife can be a good way to have a close rapport with your partner's caregivers. This is the scenario which is the least common in Australia but which gives fathers the most interaction with the caregivers involved in the birth.

This explanation is not intended to influence your decision when it comes to choosing caregivers for the birth of your baby. Rather, it is included to prepare expectant fathers for the fact that they are not necessarily given a high profile in the relationship between a birthing woman and her caregivers. I'm just giving it to you straight.

Having said that, I believe that you, the father of this child, are more important on an emotional level than any medical caregiver. You adore your partner in a way that her midwife can't. You can support her physically and emotionally in a way that no other person can. Your involvement in the birth is paramount and no one can displace you from that role. It's a big job and you need to get prepared for it.

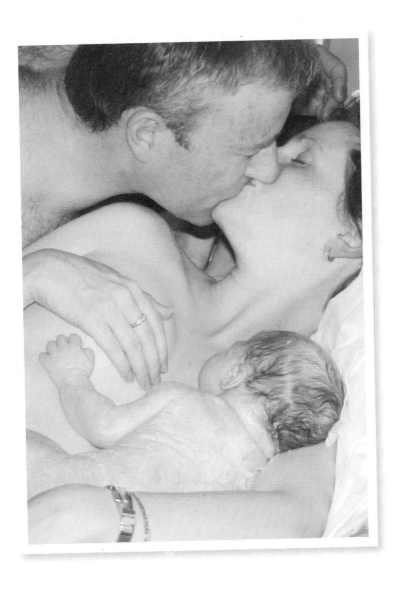

OUR BIRTH STORIES

Our first baby was born in a hospital. It was an uncomplicated birth: 12 hours prelabour and 12 hours active labour. Bang on average for a first birth. We'd been married for eight years before we started having children and I'd spent those eight years trying to convince Bruce that we should adopt. I was so afraid of childbirth that I was hoping to avoid it altogether. I really wanted to be a mother and I knew Bruce would be a ripper dad, but he wasn't interested in adoption in the slightest.

I remember an argument where I said, 'Fine! We'll have babies when you can give birth to them!' and Bruce, somewhat defeated said, 'Then why did I spend a year building this bloody big family home?' That broke my heart, so in the end I got pregnant and figured we'd deal with the whole birth part as it happened.

It wasn't until my third trimester that I realised that there was an alternative to a medically managed, medicated birth. I'd originally figured I'd have an early epidural and bypass all the agony of childbirth. I was 30 years old and 30 weeks pregnant, on a pregnancy retreat in Byron Bay when I heard my first positive, empowering birth stories. I also heard about doulas and the positive impact they can have on the birth process.

I'd left home for my Byron experience saying to Bruce, 'I won't let the hippies talk me out of an epidural!' Well, the two retreat hosts didn't try to talk me out of it, they just told me about the alternative: natural birth. I came home from Byron with a frangipani behind my ear, wanting a water birth. What a pushover!

Bruce was the best support person. He was happy to support my wishes when I wanted a medicated birth and then when I changed the game plan, he was right on board, eager to learn and willing to help. He was just so thrilled that we were starting a family at last, he'd have done anything for me.

My pregnancies were all truly HIDEOUS and each pregnancy was worse than the last. I had terrible morning sickness, awful heartburn, swollen ankles like some kind of elephant woman and a general bad mood that hung about for all three trimesters. When I met people who raved about how they looooved being pregnant, I wanted to poke them in the eye. Bruce put up with the lot. He even apologised for putting me through it.

I went into labour with Hudson a week before my due date. All three of my babies came early and I think I love them that little bit extra for putting me out of my misery sooner rather than later. I had 12 hours of prelabour, stoppy-starty contractions that didn't really hurt much, before an acupuncture treatment really got the show on the road.

Contractions were five minutes apart and lasting a full minute by the time I really needed Bruce's full attention to help me manage active labour. Before that he was packing for hospital, charging camera batteries and putting on loads of washing while I sat bouncing on a birth ball, calling out orders and timing my contractions.

For a good solid seven hours, Bruce helped me manage the labour in a very hands-on way. He was heating up heat packs in the microwave, rubbing my back, timing contractions, giving me sips of water, calling the hospital, fielding any phone calls, staring into my eyes, *ahhhhing* with me, kissing me and telling me he was so proud of me. He was busy and involved.

Our doula arrived about six hours into the active labour stage and then we made the move to hospital. Arriving at the local hospital put the brakes on my labour for a while. I was having my baby through the team midwife program and the one and only midwife I was hoping to avoid happened to be the one on shift the night I gave birth.

Darn it. Everything I wanted was denied. No, I couldn't use my birth ball. No, I couldn't use my heat packs. No, Bruce couldn't use the toilet in the birth suite. Why? Because of the threat of cross contamination, the midwife told us. Bruce and I had shared body fluids before – that's why we were here! Nonetheless, he had to walk to the other side of the hospital to use the toilet. I just had to ignore all the road blocks and get comfortable so I could birth my baby. Labour re-established once I got my rhythm back, but I think the transfer to hospital probably added a couple of hours to the whole event.

The pain was full on. No two ways about it. But it was more manageable than I had expected. The contractions responded to our pain management techniques really well. Bruce was instrumental in helping me to manage the pain. I could not have coped as well as I did without him by my side.

Once I was ten centimetres dilated and ready to push, the hard work was all up to me and I found the next two hours of pushing incredibly challenging, wishing Bruce could do some of it for me and let me have a little nap. Eventually, the midwife threatened to use the 'salad tongs' if I didn't produce this baby quickly and that gave me all the inspiration I needed to push him out! Man, did I push. The old watermelon analogy was about right.

We didn't know what gender we were having and it was such a thrill to discover our baby boy. He lay on the floor in front of us, very still and 'flat' in midwife-speak. He was quickly whipped away and given oxygen and some other medical attention.

'That was a really frightening moment,' says Bruce. 'I thought Hudson was dead. He was blue and still and the midwives wouldn't reassure us that everything was OK. They just concentrated on looking after him.'

I was in a daze, too exhausted to respond to the urgency of it all, but before too long Hudson was given the OK and brought back to us. Bruce burst into tears. Hudson's umbilical cord had been wrapped tightly around his neck, which had reduced his oxygen supply towards the end of the birth and this had made him blue and flat. He recovered quickly though and we spent a couple of hours just marvelling at our amazing little child.

'Something I wasn't ready for when Hudson was born was the amount of blood involved,' says Bruce. 'It turned out to be mainly amniotic fluid but it looked like a murder scene all over that hospital room. I wish I had been more prepared for that!'

Had we known how good Hudson's birth was going to be, we'd have had him at home. Apart from the cord drama, which is a common occurrence, his birth was easier than I had expected. But I didn't have the guts to face the unknown at home the first time and neither did Bruce. I didn't know what the pain was going to be like and wasn't totally sure that I'd be able to manage without drugs, but Hudson's birth was manageable and uncomplicated, so when I became pregnant with our second child, it was at home that I wanted to give birth.

I also carry around a fair amount of baggage when it comes to hospitals. When I was 18, I had a motorcycle accident on the approach to the Sydney Harbour Bridge. I had 14 reconstructive operations to put my leg back together and a year in plaster, all of which developed a healthy dislike of hospitals in me. To me, hospital is where I'd go if I were sick or injured. I wanted to have my babies where I was happy and healthy.

Bruce wasn't convinced about birthing at home until he asked our midwife what level of complication she could handle at home. She said, 'You don't get it. I don't do complication at home. If things start to look complicated we transfer to hospital.' So birth at home we did.

This is in no way a judgement of others and their birth choices, nor is this a recommendation that you should birth at home. I'm just telling our story and how we came to make the choice we did.

Our second child, Harlow, was born two weeks before her due date.

We have a Christmas party each year for family, friends and neighbours. Sure enough, it was on the night of our annual Christmas party that she decided to arrive. She's been the life of the party ever since.

When guests started to arrive at about 6.30pm, so did the first contractions. I had a party to run for 70 people and Santa arriving within the hour, so I just kept up the hostess act until contractions became too strong to talk through. I thought I would have hours before things got intense, but by 7.15pm I was almost ready to give birth!

I remember standing in our kitchen, with more guests pouring in by the minute, talking to our friend Greg. He asked me a question but I couldn't answer him as a contraction took over. I just leant on the kitchen bench, swayed my hips and growled. Poor Greg!

The last thing I did before I disappeared into the bathroom was to crank up the volume on the stereo so I could holler if I needed to. I caught Bruce's attention and he set about getting the sausage sizzle underway before he followed me into the bathroom, just in time to catch our daughter.

The only other person who knew what was happening was my friend Melinda. By this time, she was on the phone to Akal, our midwife, to let her know that things were progressing very fast. Melinda sat with me while I stomped my feet in the bath and when I said, 'I have to push!' she said laughing, 'Not until the midwife gets here you won't!' Melinda and I had been Girl Guides together but this night topped all our previous adventures!

I had only three pushing contractions. The first I tried to resist. With the second my waters went POP! And at the third, Harlow's head popped out. Akal was on her way but wouldn't make it for the birth so Bruce would have to catch our bub.

Meanwhile, Santa was climbing over our back fence saying, 'Ho! Ho! Ho!' and the stereo was pounding out *My Sherona*!

I'm not making this up.

Hudson was two and a half years old by then and was having the time of his life with his buddies in his new cubby house, with no idea of what we were up to in the bathroom.

Harlow's body slipped out on the next push and Bruce caught her like an expert. As Bruce has always said of this moment in his short career as an impromptu midwife, 'Bowled Mum, caught Dad!'

Bruce staggered out into the party with vernix on his T shirt and a smear of blood on his arm, killed the music and announced to everyone that his baby daughter had just been born.

The invitation had said: 'Lucy promises not to give birth on the night', so most people thought it was a joke. Then Bruce asked someone to find a bowl for the placenta and the penny dropped. The crowd went wild! Hudson came running into the bathroom and said, 'Mum, there's a baby in the bath!' then toddled off to play with his buddies.

Akal arrived and helped me birth the placenta, cut the cord and repair my tear. Darn it! The one thing I had wanted to avoid was a tear but Harlow just came out like a rocket.

Akal had put her surgical instruments in a large pot of boiling water on the stove to sterilise them. One of our party guests, thinking there might be something tasty in the pot, lifted the lid and was more than a little surprised to find a kidney dish, surgical scissors and clamps bubbling away.

Eventually, I got dressed in my party outfit again, bundled up my baby and went out to have a glass of champagne with our friends and family.

What a birth. We couldn't have planned it better if we'd tried. It really was a fabulous way to welcome a baby to the world: with all our best friends, neighbours and family who will never forget the Perry Christmas party of 2005! We like to say that the name Harlow means party crasher.

After everyone eventually went home, Bruce and I cuddled with our new little one and scoffed chocolate brownies in bed until about 2am, giggling about what had just happened.

When it came to our third, we birthed at home again. We just held off on sending out invitations.

Sheba's birth was wonderful. My pregnancy had been truly hideous, so the birth was like the gateway to a new life where I might just feel human again. My waters broke on a Friday two weeks before my due date. The following day nothing more had happened and I was in a stinking mood because this pregnancy was still persisting. I was no fun to live with.

On Sunday morning, I woke up at 9am and by 10.30am our baby girl was in my arms.

Her labour was ferociously intense. As soon as I knew I was in labour, Bruce clicked into gear, called a neighbour to look after the kids and called Akal to come *quickly*! He ran the bath and pulled out the heat packs, flicked on the music, closed the blinds, camera at the ready.

Akal knew I would go into labour at any minute and had even slept in her car outside our house on the Friday night, so she arrived like a shot, determined not to miss the birth of this one. After Harlow's rocket launcher birth, we knew that Sheba would arrive after a quick labour.

The kids thought this was a hoot! Hudson and Harlow jumped on the bed to the Beach Boys and decided that the baby should be named Tiko after the skunk in Dora the Explorer, while I paced around the bed *oooohing* and *ahhhing*.

I got into the bath for the most intense contractions while the kids watched from the end of the bath. Between contractions we talked about how it was good pain and that Mummy was all OK and that we'd be a family of five soon. They *ahhhed* with me and thought the noises I was making were really funny. The contractions were soon so intense that I felt like I had to scramble to stay ahead of them, but there were really only about five shockers before it was time to push.

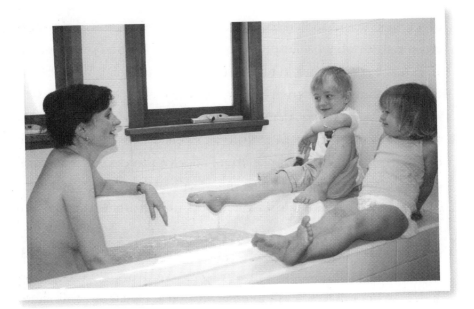

I climbed onto our bed and lay on my side with Bruce rubbing my back. A couple of plastic drop sheets from the hardware store had been thrown over the bed with towels on top to catch the mess.

Akal was guiding my pushing and my friend and neighbour Bron was holding my hand. She had come over to look after the kids but was dragged into our bedroom to help when I needed an extra hand to hold. One quick phone call and Bron's mum came over to keep an eye on Hudson and Harlow. The whole birthing saga had become a little boring for them so they were playing in their paddle pool outside.

I was conscious that Bron, in her early twenties and yet to have her own babies, didn't need to witness a horror story so having her there stopped me from screaming like a lunatic during the last couple of burning pushes. I tried not to break her fingers as well!

Three pushes and Sheba was born. We laid her next to me and I inhaled that gorgeous vernix smell that I wish I could bottle. I just kept saying, 'Isn't she beautiful?'

'Another girl!' Bruce announced with such pride. The kids came charging in and Harlow immediately tried to feed her new sister some Vegemite toast. Sheba was perfect. Almost four kilos and just beautiful, from top to toe.

Bron took the kids to church around the corner where my mum is the pastor and when they walked in she stopped the service, saying, 'Do you have something to tell us?' and Hudson said, 'Mummy's had a baby girl!' The congregation applauded and Mum burst into tears.

Akal stayed for the day, Mum came over and made us lunch and the kids welcomed their new baby sister with drawings and kisses.

When asked what the best thing was about being at the births of his sisters, Hudson, aged five, said, 'It was just so cool that they were born out of your tummy and I could see them straight away. They were so little and beautiful. I couldn't stop kissing them. I wish we could have another one.'

So do I!

CHAPTER 2

CALL FOR REINFORCEMENTS

Many men find the role of childbirth support partner to be quite overwhelming and feel the need for support for themselves, never mind needing to be a pillar of strength for their partner. The average first birth involves 12 to 18 hours of active labour (not to mention prelabour which can go on for days). This is a long time to be the sole emotional and physical support person for the birthing mother.

A doula is a professionally trained childbirth support person or birth attendant, who gives physical and emotional support as well as unbiased information to the birthing couple. She can help you feel more relaxed, confident and emotionally available to your partner. A good doula is unobtrusive, compassionate and non-judgemental. She shouldn't talk too much and she certainly shouldn't try to influence your choices.

A doula does not replace the midwives or an obstetrician, nor does a doula have a clinical role in the birth. She is like a hired friend who happens to have a lot of experience in childbirth, has generally had babies of her own and is passionate about supporting expectant parents as they welcome their little one into the world.

'I wanted a doula to support me as well as my wife during the birth of our son,' says Bruce. 'I didn't know how long the birth was going to last and didn't feel comfortable being my partner's only support person. What if I lost the plot? What if I got totally exhausted and let her down? Having a doula made me feel more confident to participate in the birth. And she made me coffee!'

Many expectant couples are surprised to find that they will spend great slabs of time all alone during a hospital birth. Unless there is a medical reason for constantly monitoring the labour, the midwives will leave you alone for the majority of the time, checking in on you briefly every hour or so, only staying with you if you feel you need help. Only when the pushing stage commences and the birth is imminent will a midwife stay with you continuously and right at the end, another midwife may join you as well to see to the safe delivery of the baby.

If you have private healthcare, the obstetrician will be contacted by the midwives during labour and called in towards the end, usually once the birthing mother starts to push. The obstetrician will arrive for the exciting part, deliver the baby, then leave you to it.

While the average first labour lasts 12 to 18 hours, a standard midwifery shift is 8 hours during the day and 10 hours at night. With this in mind, there is a good chance that the labour will go through a shift change, your caregiver will go home and you'll have a new midwife assigned to your birth. A birthing woman becomes very attached to her support team and the change in caregivers can be disconcerting and can change the rhythm that she has become dependent on. On the other hand, she might feel that she and her midwife haven't really gelled and the shift change might be welcome.

Having a doula gives both you and your partner continuity of support from labouring at home, to the hospital environment and through hospital shift changes. The comings and goings of midwives matter a whole lot less when you have a doula with you all the way through.

'With our system the way it is, doulas have become an absolute necessity,' says Associate Professor of Midwifery, Hannah Dahlen.

'This problem is not due to lack of health funding, it's because the health system treats pregnancy and birth as an illness,' says Hannah. 'Instead of treating only the necessary cases as medical events, we intervene in many more cases than we should and this absorbs midwifery resources to the point that midwives can't always fulfil the role that doulas do.'

Studies[1] have shown that women who have the support of a doula have shorter labours, fewer medical interventions, fewer Caesareans and healthier babies. Evidence also suggests that women who have a doula have a more satisfying birth experience and fewer problems with breastfeeding and bonding.

Too good to be true? The studies referred to above have shown that the presence of a doula reduces:

- the overall Caesarean rate by 45%
- the length of labour by 25%
- Syntocinon use by 50%
- pain medication by 31%
- need for assisted deliveries by 34%
- requests for epidurals by up to 60%
- problems with breastfeeding and bonding

What about dads and doulas? A doula certainly doesn't replace the role of the dad. No one can love the birthing mother like her partner can and she will need you close to her when she is giving birth.

'A father's fear is reduced enormously when he knows he has a doula's support,' says birth attendant Denise Love, who has attended over four thousand births over the last three decades. 'Some men are terrified of having a big blow up with their partner. They've heard from their men friends that their partner will scream and swear and spend the rest of her life telling him he didn't support her properly through childbirth. Women have very high expectations of their men when they give birth.'

Denise says that doulas are like stage directors. They're in the background helping the dad support his partner in all the right ways.

When I visit a couple after their birth and the mother tells me that she couldn't have done it without her husband and, 'Didn't he do a great job?' then I know I've done my job well. I've helped her husband to be the support person she needed him to be, without being overly obvious about it.

'There are three key factors that influence a woman in labour,' says Dr John Keogh: 'One-to-one nursing care, mobilisation during labour and having experienced, knowledgeable, female support such as a doula. Doulas can also help reassure fathers that everything is OK and that the birth process is normal. Every little variation can seem a big problem when you don't know exactly what's happening and the doula can help interpret what is going on.'

You can expect to pay several hundred dollars or more for a doula, depending on her experience and the length of time she spends with you before and after the birth. Some doulas charge thousands but this fee may include professional services such as prenatal massage or acupuncture. The usual doula's fee includes spending some time with you as a couple before the birth to get to know your birth wishes. It also includes attending the birth – for as long as it takes – as well as a postnatal visit and debrief.

If the budget won't allow for additional support, you can hire a student doula for little or no cost. Doulas-in-training are required to attend three or more births during their course. You may also be asked to fill in feedback forms as part of their assessment and you may be phoned or emailed by their tutor. Just be aware that you may have a trainee on her very first birth, a possibility which comes with the territory.

You should like your doula from the minute you meet her. You are inviting her into a very special occasion and she should fit in well with you as a couple. Most importantly, make sure that your doula is there to support your birthing wishes and is not trying to push you down any particular path of her own choosing.

'It is not a doula's role to tell a woman how to give birth,' says Perth doula trainer, childbirth educator and mother of two, Cath Cook. 'Rather, it is the doula's role to help the expectant couple to understand their options in order to decide how they want to give birth.'

Cath emphasises that couples come to birth with different life experiences and these will shape their choices surrounding childbirth. A good doula respects her clients without judgement and will support them in their decisions, whatever they may be.

Make sure your doula has been thoroughly trained for the task and is happy to support you in your wishes, without interfering in any way with your partner's medical care. Run a mile from a doula who says you should birth a certain way or who comes with a combative approach to your caregivers. Avoid a doula who charges by the hour – your partner doesn't want to worry that a long labour is going to cost a fortune.

There are also postnatal doulas who work with new parents to help them with the transition into parenthood on a practical level. This can include helping with breastfeeding issues and settling techniques as well as taking care of cooking, housework and looking after other children.

To find a birth doula or postnatal doula in your area, visit *www.findadoula.com.au*. I established this website a few years ago so that doulas could make themselves known to their community and so that couples could find a doula to support them. The search function is free to use and after the birth you can leave feedback about your doula for others to read.

Other support people

Women need to feel totally uninhibited to give birth freely and naturally. When you invite family members or friends to the birth, they bring with them their own childbirth baggage and the relationship baggage that they might have with you and your partner.

Your partner needs to feel totally free to birth with confidence. Think carefully before you invite friends, sisters and especially your mother or your partner's mother to the birth of your child.

Denise Love, who has a Masters in nursing, tells this story: 'I attended a birth where the woman had said to her partner, "Number one, under no circumstances is your mother to come to the hospital while I'm having this baby. Number two, you have to turn your phone off the minute I go into labour." He was a mummy's boy and his mum was likely to call 600 times during the labour so it was obvious that he just wouldn't be able to ignore those phone calls, but he agreed to his partner's terms. During the birth, sure enough, his phone rings and he disappears without telling his partner. He comes back half an hour later with his mother in tow. The marriage ended and it was partly because of that betrayal.'

One of the most common questions that I'm asked by expectant dads is about their mother-in-law. The question usually goes something like this: *My wife has asked her mother to be at the birth. She thinks her mum would like to be there but I think this should be just between us as a couple. What if my mother-in-law starts calling the shots?*

The best approach to this common dilemma is to have a heart-to-heart with your partner. Ask her if she really can't imagine giving birth without her mother by her side. If this is the case, then your mother-in-law needs to be there, but if your partner is not sure, it's better not to have her mother present. If your partner has invited her mum to be there for her *mother's* sake, this is not a good idea. It takes a very unique mother-daughter relationship to have the grandmother of the child in an active role at the birth.

'Some mothers are wonderful support partners for their daughters, especially if they have a good relationship with their son-in-law,' says John Keogh. However, Dr Keogh has seen some situations where the grandparents have not behaved well. 'When I was a registrar, I was looking after a woman in labour who was progressing very well when in stormed her mother-in-law. This big, commanding woman physically picked up the midwife and put her on the other side of the room, then marched to her daughter-in-law's bedside and slapped her in the face! I couldn't believe what was happening.'

I know of a birth where the woman's mother was in attendance. The labouring woman had a touchy relationship with her mother and had invited her to the birth as a gesture of peace. This was a mistake. Her mother was emotionally unavailable, critical of the way her daughter wanted to birth (which was loud with lots of swearing) and hampered her daughter's progress with her obvious disapproval. After hours and hours of this, the woman eventually asked her mother to leave. Within an hour, she had given birth. This woman needed the freedom to birth the way she wanted to and having her mother and all that mother-daughter baggage in the room was detrimental to her progress.

Another birth I attended was with a couple having their second child. When they had given birth to their first, his mother-in-law had been present. Back when she had given birth it had been with nuns in attendance and she'd been told to birth in silence. So when it came to her grandchild's birth, all the huffing and puffing and *ahhhing* really bothered her. She spent the entire birth patting her daughter's shoulder, telling her to *shhhhhhhh*. When I came to support this couple to have their second child, this time with no mother present, the brief was to let her holler as loud as she needed to and wow, did she shout the house down! It was great. She just needed the freedom to do what she wanted without her mother's childbirth baggage interfering. It was the most uncomplicated, easy birth I think I've ever attended.

Our mothers gave birth in a different era. They were told to keep quiet, to lie on their back and submit to medical management. Your partner is birthing in a time where women freely shout the house down, call the shots in the birth suite and feel free to ask for crazy things like bean bags and mirrors. Let her have the freedom to do this without her mother's judgement.

'Mothers and sisters just shouldn't be at births,' says Denise Love, who doesn't pull her punches. 'Sisters dump on their sisters. They can say things like, "Oh, you always were a whinger," or they say to me, "She's been a drama queen since we were kids!" And it's often the sister who hasn't had any kids who's saying this!'

'I've been asked by so many women to tell their mother to leave the birth suite. I remember a woman who came to her daughter's birth in her clippety-clop high heels, with gold bangles jangling on her arms: hardly prepared for the hard work of supporting a woman through natural childbirth. The daughter looked at me and even though she had asked her mother to be there, said to me, "Get my mother the hell out of here!" I had to say, "Thanks so much for coming, I'll call you when we need you."'

If your mother-in-law is a midwife, you're in trouble. She'll want to be there for the birth of your child because this is her profession, her daughter and her grandchild!

'Even if your mother-in-law is the Dalai Lama, she shouldn't be at the birth of her grandchild,' says Denise. 'She's in a position of power over the father of the child, even more so if she's also a midwife.'

Apart from mothers, some women like to have their sister or a girlfriend in attendance. Think about what these other people will be bringing to the birth. If her sister or girlfriend has had four children, well then she brings experience. But remember, she brings her childbirth baggage with her too. Will she be supporting your partner to birth the way she wants to or the way you as a couple want to? This is a conversation you should have with this person if she is to attend the birth. How will you work together? Who calls the shots once your partner has lost her sense of humour? Will this person be willing to leave if you ask her to? These are important things to clarify if you invite others to the birth.

I had a group attend one of my pub workshops once: the pregnant woman, her husband and her two oldest girlfriends. The two friends had never given birth, they were just along for the ride. Over dinner, I asked them what they thought their role would be in this birth. One of them said, 'To make sure he turns up!' and pointed to the expectant dad. Neither of them had a clue how to help their friend through the birth, they just thought it would be fun to watch. By the end of the workshop, when they had a clearer picture of what childbirth can be like and what would be expected of them, they weren't so jovial. They realised that there was a big job to do and that if they didn't support their friend properly, they could actually make the labour slower and more painful for her. I never did hear how that birth went.

> *To summarise, if you really want to know what I think, let it be just you, your partner and if you can afford it, an experienced doula. No extra spectators.*

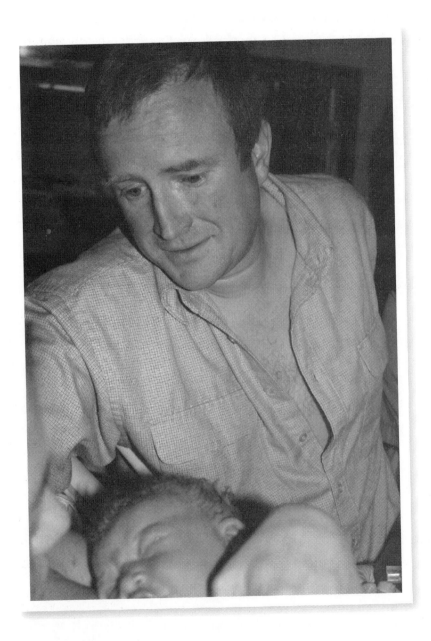

PAUL TRESEDER'S STORY

I was shocked by the sudden urge of protective anger for my woman.

Paul Treseder has been flying planes since he was 16 years old. He is from a flying family, his father a pilot and his mother a 'hostie'. For the last 15 years, Paul has flown jumbos on long haul routes for Qantas, initially as First Officer and now as Captain. He now flies domestic routes so that he can see more of his wife Lucy Barker, an accomplished artist, and their young children Ted and Lola. Paul was on the ground when Ted was born by emergency Caesarean and together the couple brought in the help of a doula (or birth attendant) for Lola's birth. Here Paul tells it as only a pilot can…

I met my wife Lucy at a party in 2002. We didn't really date, our paths just converged and we were together from then on. It was soon after we met that I flew her to Rome with me. Italians always applaud a smooth landing, so perhaps my landing the plane to a round of applause helped to win her over.

The longest straight flight is the Melbourne to LA route, which is 16 hours. That route is an exercise in fatigue management because you have to be able to deliver at the pointy end of the trip. The birth of Ted was similar in that it was long and tiring and at the pointy end, I had to be there for Lucy.

We really wanted a natural birth for Ted but the cascade of intervention began within 24 hours of Lucy's waters breaking. My biggest regret for Ted's birth is that I didn't negotiate harder for more time to let the labour start spontaneously.

In an aircraft, passengers are not encouraged to assist the flight crew.

In the hospital environment, I gave the medical team the professional respect I felt they deserved. However, there was a case once where a passenger (granted, he was a pilot) noticed ice on a wing and mentioned it to the flight attendant. She didn't pass on the information to the captain and the plane crashed. In retrospect, as a 'passenger' on this birth trip perhaps I could have spoken up sooner and tried harder to avoid the interventions that led to the Caesarean.

Lucy was put on a Syntocinon drip to start the labour and very quickly the pain hit the roof.

I was aware that I was required to be useful during this stage. I'm not sure that I actually was but I was certainly trying very hard. We used various active childbirth techniques. The most effective tool in our bag of tricks was a ball that we threw to each other and we played catch to distract her from the pain. Unfortunately, we had a midwife who had just come back to work after a trip to Vietnam and all she wanted to talk about was her trip. I thought the midwife would help with the pain management but all she did was tell us about her holiday.

Lucy tried the nitrous oxide gas but this didn't help her much so within four hours of the induction, she was asking for an epidural. She was suffering tremendously so we went ahead with the next intervention. Lucy was tired and had some rest while I did the cryptic crossword, something I've completed only about 20 times in my whole life. I was stuck on one of the questions and there was the nitrous oxide by the bed. I tried the gas and it magically cleared my head! Every time I got stuck I had a little gas and I finished the crossword in record time: at least some good came of the nitrous oxide.

After a few hours, they told us that our baby was in distress and that we had to have a Caesarean. Lucy is a no-fuss girl and she adapted to the idea quickly but she was scared. This was not the birth we had hoped for.

Fear is contagious. As pilot, you remain calm so that everyone else remains calm. I'll never forget an incident years ago when I was a fairly new second officer (something like an apprentice airline pilot). A flight attendant called the flight deck shortly after takeoff to report sparks and flames in one of the engines. The captain said with perfect calm, 'Paul, would you mind looking out the window for me and telling me what you see?' I did and I could report that there were in fact sparks and flames in the fourth engine.

There have been cases when a fire on board has gone from detection of smoke to a ditched plane within 14 minutes, so a fire on board is a very serious matter. You must act promptly.

The captain said with a casual sense of calm and control, 'That is a disappointment isn't it?' We shut down the engine, dumped 130 odd thousand kilos of fuel in the Gulf of Siam and returned to land. To me, that was how a captain behaved: calm and with no sign of fear whatsoever.

I wanted to be calm for Lucy and didn't want to show her any fear as we faced surgery. From the time the decision was made to have the operation to the incision itself, was only about 20 minutes.

Theatre was a very weird environment. A midwife said to me in a stern manner, 'That's your chair. Sit in it and don't move.' I thought, 'They must get some real psychos in here if they have to control us like that.'

Then the doctors pulled on the incision with their hands to really open her up and I suddenly had an overwhelming urge to thump the men operating on my wife. I was shocked by the sudden urge of protective anger for my woman. The primal, lizard bit of the brain had taken the wheel!

When Ted was born, Lucy seemed more relieved that it was over than pleased to see her baby, to be honest. She says she was full of pethidine and doesn't really remember it. There's a famous family photo of Lucy and Ted and she looks peaceful, happy and overjoyed. I was just so happy to have a child but I felt torn between leaving Lucy in theatre and taking my boy to the ward.

Long haul pilots greet each other in terms of sleep. 'Get some sleep?' or 'Are you rested?' they might say to their crew at the start of a trip. It's a traditional long haul topic. Before I became a father, I'd never looked at long haul as a means of getting rest. It's an exhausting job. But once we had Ted, I got more rest when I was away on long haul than when I was at home. I stopped going for drinks with the boys and would head straight to my hotel for sleep. Pilots wake up, look at the time and count how many hours they've slept. At home I often didn't have very many to count. Ted was always an active boy with an enquiring mind and has turned out to be such a lovely chap, but those early days were *very* tiring.

Within a couple of days of falling pregnant the second time, Lucy and I were discussing the idea of having a doula at our next birth. It's a pity we didn't know about doulas the first time.

The second birth was a lot less dramatic. We were aiming for a spontaneous labour as we knew a second Caesarean would mean Caesareans for all future births. We got to know our doula and she became part of the birth team. Lucy and I made the decisions but our doula was part of the information process. We used our active childbirth bag of tricks again. It was the vanilla birth we were hoping for. All natural, lots of pain, pretty quick. At one point during pushing I had my arm under Lucy's head and she went for me and tried to bite me!

After each of the births I was filled with admiration for my wife.

I really value having kids for the change in perspective that it has given me. In fact, becoming a father has made me a better pilot. I have a heightened sense of responsibility. That first departure when I left Lucy and Ted to go back to flying, I remember looking out the window of the taxi and feeling a great sense of satisfaction. I wasn't just building a career, flying jets. I was providing for a family now.

CHAPTER 3

WHAT TO SAY AND WHAT NOT TO SAY DURING CHILDBIRTH

Pregnant, labouring and lactating women are very sensitive and your words are powerful. If you come into contact with a woman who is pregnant, in labour or postpartum, remember that you have the power to make her day or break her heart. Think about your tone, your words and any judgements you may be inadvertently passing. Simple language that you use every day has extra weight with a woman in labour.

When you are supporting a woman through childbirth, you may have to behave a little out of character to support her effectively. For example, if you're usually the life of the party, this is the one day in your life that you may need to SHUT UP. As a doula, that's my constant challenge because I can talk under wet cement. Every time I open my mouth when I'm beside a labouring woman, I think, 'Do I really need to say this, or am I just talking for the sake of it?'

I remember supporting a lovely couple who were having their third child. He was a great guy, really chatty and totally into his wife. When it came to the birth, do you think we could shut him up? He was thrilled that the baby would be born at night. He'd been fretting about the timing because he was a dentist and what would happen if he'd just started a three-hour procedure when his wife went into labour? Third babies usually come quite fast and their second had been a very fast labour. When his wife went into labour in the evening, all the pressure was off and he was so relieved, he was having the time of his life! He was yacking all the way through her contractions, high-fiving the obstetrician and flirting with the midwives. He was just so thrilled! This took attention away from the birthing mother and meant she had to work hard to ignore him and stay focused as she laboured. Finally, she said through gritted teeth, 'Will you shut up!'

It's easy to make the mistake of being a motor mouth because you're excited about the imminent birth and there is also a lot of time to pass. It's tempting to fill the silence by chatting to the midwives and chumming up to the obstetrician.

However, too much talk will slow her labour down. When a woman is in labour, she is using the ancient, primal part of the brain. This part of the brain directs our instinctive behaviour and labour is essentially a natural instinct. To labour effectively, she needs to be able to use this primal part of her brain as much as possible. Language skills are governed by a much more recent development in the brain, the neocortex. If you are engaging in too much language with your partner, you stimulate the neocortex, which will effectively interfere with your partner's natural instinct and slow down her labour. So limit the amount you talk and especially the number of questions you ask her.

Do you want a drink? What about a pillow? Would you like to be in the bath? On the bed? Shall I call the midwife? Want a muesli bar? Where are the CDs? What did I do with my phone?

Just decide if she needs a pillow, just call the midwife. Use your common sense. You will relieve your partner of the decision-making she doesn't have the brain capacity to deal with at the time and prevent her from having to think too much and talk too much herself.

I had a dad at one of my workshops whose mother-in-law was a midwife and was flying in from Europe to attend the birth. The mother-in-law spoke only Spanish while he spoke English and French. His partner could speak English and Spanish. This meant that the labouring woman was going to have to translate between her two support people. This was a bad idea. She would have had to engage the neocortex throughout her labour just to facilitate communication between her husband and her mother!

My friend Mika is Japanese and says that when she is tired, she loses her fluency in English. Before she went into labour, she asked her Australian husband to speak for her so that she could concentrate on birthing rather than on her spoken English. As it turned out, Mika discovered that her body language and her caregiver's ability to read her body language were far more important than verbal translation of what was going on. 'In a way, it's like going back to being "animal" without spoken language,' says Mika. 'Mika's body language included nearly biting my finger in half!' says her husband Peter. 'Men need to understand what a primal process childbirth is.'

Don't talk during contractions and don't tolerate it from staff. You need to be totally focused on helping your partner through each contraction, so chatting to the midwife is a distraction that is not helpful.

On the other hand, you might be a pretty quiet chap and your partner may usually be the one who speaks up if something is to be said. While she's in labour, especially towards the end, she won't be able to call the shots. She'll need you to be the spokesperson for your family and speak up when she needs you to.

One of the longest births I've ever attended was with a lovely, quiet, friendly couple. She was not going to have an epidural no matter what and worked very hard to manage without one for many hours. Her birth plan had been very specific: no drugs. At seven in the morning after we'd been at it for about 20 hours, a resident doctor breezed in, fresh as a daisy, offering an epidural. None of us had even said the word epidural out loud before then! As the doula, I'm there thinking about what to say, when the dad stepped in with quiet confidence.

'We have a birth plan in place,' he said. 'Have you had a chance to read it?' The doctor hadn't, which is to be expected. 'We are doing extremely well and my wife has requested not to have any drugs offered whatsoever. You may leave us to manage this alone. Are there any questions?'

He handled the doctor so well. For a bloke of few words, he said exactly the right thing when it was necessary.

Mind your language

The technical language of childbirth is sometimes negative. Terms such as 'incompetent cervix' and 'failure to progress' are common terms used by medical professionals, but they are words that can have a negative effect on the birthing mother and can make her feel like a failure before she's even begun.

Women need to feel safe and supported to be able to open up and let go but they can't do this if they are being told that they are a failure. It's like cheering on your marathon runner on the side-lines and yelling, 'You're so damn slow, you big failure!'

There are many obstetric terms that don't do women in labour any favours. Apparently I have an 'irritable uterus' and some women are less than thrilled to hear that they are 'failing to dilate'.

Leave the negative obstetric language to the professionals (who need to communicate with a common technical language) and keep your own language positive and empowering for the woman who is hanging on your every word.

Don't complain about your own aches and pains

This might seem like an obvious tip but it's very commonly overlooked. Childbirth can take a long, long time and it can get dead boring. Your back can ache, your bum goes numb, your fingers turn to prunes in the shower. It doesn't matter. Your pain and suffering is of no consequence in the birth of your baby and should never be mentioned. It's fair to say that the birthing mother is in significantly more discomfort than you are at that moment in time.

Be alert, not alarmed

If you like a drink or two you're likely to enjoy several months of having a designated driver in the family, with most pregnant women avoiding alcohol altogether. However, by about the 37-week mark, expectant fathers really need to be on call to attend the birth 24 hours a day. This means you need to be 100% sober, 100% of the time once your baby's due date is approaching. When I was about 36 weeks pregnant with my first, I had a false alarm with some powerful contractions for a few hours. We'd had an afternoon entertaining friends and Bruce had had a few beers – too many to drive safely – so we had to ask a neighbour to drive us to the hospital for what we thought was going to be the birth of our baby. Bruce was so embarrassed that he couldn't fulfil this basic task when I needed him to. From then on he made sure that he could drive at any time of the day or night.

This also means taking care with medications, especially the heavily sedating kind. My friend Sue gave birth to her third baby on the couch at home, while her husband Graeme was overseas. The baby arrived nearly four weeks early, when her first two had been overdue, so she and Graeme were understandably taken by surprise. When Sue went into labour, her mother-in-law was sleeping soundly in the spare room after taking two sleeping pills. The older children slept while Sue, in active labour, tried unsuccessfully to wake her sedated mother-in-law. Sue laboured alone while her mum came racing across town, calling an ambulance on the way and walking in the door only a few minutes before the baby was born. Sue's mother-in-law had finally woken up and the two grandmothers were there to catch the baby, with only minutes to spare.

The moral to this story is that you need to be alert to look after your partner when she has this baby, not over the limit or sedated.

Denise Love tells a story of a dad she supported, who between contractions let out a big yawn and said, 'Sheesh, this is boring isn't it?'

It sounds like a throw-away comment and who else can you confide in but your beloved? However, the birthing mother hears it differently. She hears: 'I'm distracted from what you're going through. I can't relate to the pain you're in. I'm selfish and lazy. I'm bored by the miracle that is the birth of our baby. I'd rather be watching TV.'

Do not take any entertainment devices or boredom-breakers to the birth. That includes the newspaper, your laptop or a good book. You'll live.

If the worst thing that happens during this labour is that you are bored to snores, you'll have done well! There are periods of time between contractions when nothing is happening and you'll wish you could read the paper or check your emails. But you can't. You have to stay focused on your partner and attentive to her needs, which might all be boring and uncomfortable for you. Like I said, you'll live.

During the birth of our first, when it came time to push, I sat on a birth stool and Bruce sat behind me supporting me. We sat like this for a couple of hours and eventually Bruce's bum went completely numb. His advice to you is to take your wallet out of your back pocket and don't complain about the fact that you've stopped feeling your legs.

Don't compare what your partner is going through to the time you passed a gall stone or when your appendix ruptured. It's a completely different kind of pain and the analogy is of no use to your partner. She doesn't want to hear it so don't let it cross your lips.

Don't give birth a time frame

The baby doesn't know what time it is and the uterus can only work as fast as it is able so there is no point in placing time frames on birth. Don't comment on the length of time the birth is taking. Childbirth can be a very slow process, so get your head around that fact now. It's not unusual for there to be up to 24 hours of prelabour where contractions are gentle and sporadic followed by 12 to 16 hours of active labour and then two hours of pushing. You might be on duty for over 30 hours by the time your baby is born and it's usually several hours after that before your head will hit a pillow.

Those super-fast births in the backs of ambulances are generally reserved for women having their second and subsequent babies so if you are a first timer, be prepared for the long haul and be pleasantly surprised if it's a faster labour.

Take your watch off if that helps you stay focused on the birth. You can be confident that the midwives will be keeping track of the time and won't let the labour go on for so long that it threatens your baby's health.

Even putting a positive spin on the time isn't helpful. If things are moving along well and you say, 'I think we'll have this baby by lunch time,' you're inadvertently putting an expectation on your partner to perform to a time frame. When lunch time comes and goes, and so does dinner time and then you're still looking at each other when it's getting light the following morning, she may feel like a failure. This might sound over-sensitive, but then labouring women are.

There was only one time during any of my labours when there was a time frame applied to my progress. Towards the end of my son's birth, I had fully dilated, but the midwife said there was a thin cervical lip that needed some more time to efface. She suggested that we wait for half an hour and then do another internal examination before I could start pushing my baby out.

It was the longest half an hour of my entire labour. I sat there watching the clock and that stinking second hand seemed to move so slowly. If the midwife had just said that she'd come back in a little while and check on me, I'd have lost track of time, but giving me a time frame gave me an unhelpful focus.

Don't talk about anything outside the birth

Your partner needs to feel that you are concentrating on her and frankly, the world outside could stop spinning and she wouldn't care, so don't talk about anything outside the birth.

I remember a story of a woman whose husband went to get a coffee while she laboured away and when he came back he said, 'Hey, I saw Barry from our local bottle shop at the vending machine!' She said she could almost feel her cervix closing over at the thought of Barry from the bottle shop being out there in the corridor while she was buck naked, on all fours, growling through each contraction.

You are in the birth world, so stay focused on this.

I heard a story about a woman who always had long labours so she sent her husband home for some sleep while she laboured with her doula present. On the way home, he got thinking. This was their third child and they really should consider buying a bigger car. So instead of going home, he headed off to a local car dealership to check out the latest models.

A couple of hours later, he returned to the hospital with paperwork for her to sign for a brand new station wagon! She was furious and her labour completely stalled while they argued about this massive, untimely financial commitment. I'm not sure if she signed the papers, but once they had settled their argument and all car brochures and contracts had been banished from the room, her labour re-established.

You need to remain fully present for your partner and that takes some concentration. By this I don't mean just being in the room and not wandering off. I mean, you have to stay with her emotionally, stay focused on every contraction and not let yourself be distracted by anything or anyone. The buzz of all the medical machinery and the whole hospital environment might be intriguing, but don't let it distract you from the important task at hand, which is to support your partner in every way.

Look after yourself so that you can look after her

Don't faint! That might sound easy to say but if you are going to hit the deck, you will feel it coming. You'll feel light headed and dizzy and you may feel nauseous as your blood pressure suddenly drops.

The best thing to do is sit down and put your head between your knees. This lets the blood run back to your head so you won't black out. A doctor at one of my workshops once suggested that you could pretend to be tying up your shoelaces.

Stay well hydrated and sit down when you have the opportunity. There are usually plenty of stools, birth balls and chairs to sit on and no one expects you to stand the whole time. You're no good to anyone if you're taken off to have stitches in your head and you will take the emphasis away from the birthing mother if you become an emergency. If you know you are of the squeamish kind, don't go down the business end or watch stitches being done.

You'll be unpopular if you stink, so look after your personal hygiene. You've probably already noticed that your partner's sense of smell is heightened during pregnancy and it's up another notch when she's in labour. You'll be working physically hard to support your partner and this may go on for days so you'll need a clean T shirt, some breath mints and deodorant. Keep yourself nice.

Pack your swimmers if you would like to get into the bath or shower with your partner. Labouring women can get naked in the labour ward, but if you get your gear off, they'll call security. See Chapter 8 for a detailed packing list for hospital.

Our neighbour Peter has a practical tip for men who want to get into the bath with their partner: go to the toilet first. Peter's wife chose the hospital where she gave birth because the spa baths were nice and deep and this would help with her natural pain management. In the end it was Peter needing pain management as he held on for hours while his wife wouldn't let him leave her side.

As support partner, you should eat small snacks regularly as well as staying well hydrated. Food that has some protein for sustained energy is ideal and some sugar is also helpful.

'I was at a birth recently where the father kept disappearing to visit the vending machine to get a coffee and would come back with revolting coffee breath,' says birth consultant Denise Love. 'Then he sat next to his wife with a bag of chips and munched in her ear. I said to him three times, "You're going to get your head bitten off," and he said to me, "I'm hungry, I'm going to eat!"' What a turkey.

Cheese sandwiches cut into quarters are the perfect snack because they're quiet to eat. You can't be munching in your partner's ear.

Protein bars are excellent as well, giving you sustained energy over the next couple of hours and making you feel full too. Snakes or barley sugars will give you a sugar lift. Your partner will be breathing in and out of her mouth a lot, which will make her mouth manky, but some sugar will clear her tongue. Breath mints are self-explanatory, especially if you're a coffee drinker. Energy drinks are good too because they have sugar and salts in them to keep you going.

Stay positive, no matter what

Most importantly, you need to maintain a positive attitude throughout the birth. Your partner needs to know that you are proud of her, no matter what, and that you don't doubt her natural ability to give birth for one second. And she needs to know that you adore her. You are her rock and you will not help your partner get through this if you fall apart. If your birth outcome is unexpected and difficult, there is time for falling apart later, but through the labour, you have to give your partner all the positive reinforcement you can muster, no matter what.

I did my doula training with a woman who gained her doula certification just to understand birth better, but not with a view to actually attending births. I thought this was fascinating and asked her why. She had had a long, difficult labour herself and couldn't dilate beyond about three centimetres. Her husband was quite emotionally absent during the birth and wasn't able to support her the way she really needed. He was stressed out that things were not progressing as they should. The baby eventually went into distress and her obstetrician decided that he should perform an emergency Caesarean. This was the couple's greatest fear and the expectant dad fell apart. He literally burst into tears, curled up on the floor and phoned his mother.

The labouring woman felt totally abandoned by her husband. Years later she was still processing the trauma of abandonment and battling postnatal depression.

So, if your partner's already in prelabour and you left it until now to read this book, this is what you need to remember:

- *Don't talk too much*
- *Keep your language positive*
- *Don't complain about your aches and pains*
- *Don't give birth a time frame*
- *Be 100% present*
- *Don't talk about anything outside the birth*
- *Look after yourself so that you can look after her*
- *Stay positive no matter what!*

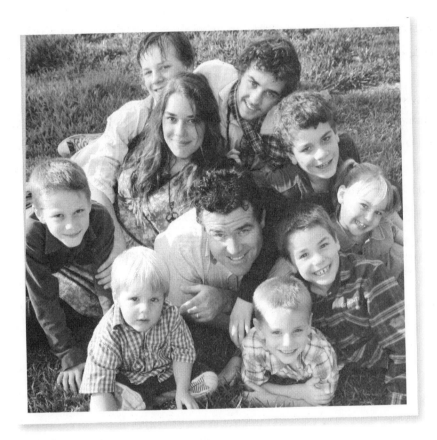

PAUL OSBORNE'S STORY

Sally's given birth every which way with our nine children: all natural, induced, with drugs for pain and without, as well as a Caesarean.

Paul Osborne is the Chief Executive Officer of the Parramatta Eels in Sydney. He's a former police detective and played rugby league for St George Illawarra Dragons and then the Canberra Raiders before spending six years in state politics in the ACT. Together with his wife Sally, they have nine children. That's right, nine. They range in age from toddlers to teenagers and all nine of them are home schooled. Paul was there for all nine births, including a Caesarean. Here is his story.

Sally had great pregnancies with no morning sickness at all. The only drama was during her eighth pregnancy when she had lots of bleeding and had to be on bed-rest. We lived on a farm near Canberra at the time so that one was a worry, but the other eight pregnancies were great.

We never intended to have nine kids. I thought we'd stop at Jacob, our second child, but I went into politics with two kids and I came out with seven. I was too busy and obviously wasn't paying attention and next thing I knew, we had a big family. I'd thought I was doing it for pleasure, not babies!

We were both 24 years old when we had our first child and I was just a young, selfish football player. I went to only one night of antenatal classes and never went back. I wasn't going to sit through all that crap.

Going into that first birth, my biggest worry was how such a big head was going to come out of such a small place. It was scary and I really didn't know what we were in for.

Sally's obstetrician was an obnoxious fool. I should have fired him from the start. He had absolutely no compassion for a woman who was giving birth for the first time. We wanted her to give birth in a hospital where she could have the option of drugs and the best medical care if she needed it, but she would have fared better with a kinder doctor.

The first birth was a long labour, about 16 hours, all natural, without any drugs for the pain. Sally was amazing. It was so raw, so exhausting. The birth was long, slow and tiring for both of us. The doctor says, 'She's dilated four centimetres,' and I'm thinking, 'Yeah? What does that mean?' I had no clue.

Sabella came out looking pretty terrible – she was all puffed up and looking pretty rough. She's gorgeous now. Sally fell in love with our children from the moment she laid eyes on each of them, but I take time to fall in love with them. I get to know them and adore them, but it's not an instant thing for me because I'm not full of birth hormones.

I 'steal' our children from Sally when they're between one and two years old. I'm like a Great White. I just circle until I think they're ready to be close to Dad and then I go in and take them and they're all mine! Five boys in a row have brushed their mother off and only have eyes for their dad! Secretly, I've told each one of my kids that they're my favourite but I'm really close to all nine of them and I love being a dad.

Life with a newborn was a big adjustment. Sally would say I wasn't very helpful at that stage of the game. I thought I knew more than she did and had a lot to say, especially when it came to breastfeeding and attachment. I saw the midwife show Sally how to do it once and then I figured I was an expert.

Dr Roger Heaton delivered the other eight babies. At the time, he delivered all the babies for the Raiders football players in Canberra. Sally and I hold the record for the number of babies born to one family at John James Hospital in Canberra. Roger's a mad St George fan and I was eventually banned from going to prenatal visits because we talked too much footy but he was really kind to Sally and he put me at ease. He mainly talked footy to distract me and keep me calm.

I was more worried with each labour, pacing the floor, observing. I was a shocker – a total pest to Roger. I wouldn't let him go home while Sally was in labour. He'd say, 'She's five centimetres dilated, I'll come back soon,' and I'd say, 'No way, if you walk out that door, she'll jump to eight centimetres!'

Sally's given birth every which way with our nine children: all natural, induced, with drugs for pain and without, as well as a Caesarean.

Our fourth child, George, was born so fast I had to be Adam Gilchrist to catch him! Then the next one, Thomas, took seven hours to arrive, so each birth was unpredictable.

The Caesarean for Daisy was scary but it all went smoothly in the end. Sally had placenta previa [where the placenta grows over the cervix, preventing the baby from being delivered naturally] and I was really worried. I'm thinking, 'I can't look after all these kids on my own!'

Being in theatre was very different after seven babies in the labour ward. It only took about ten minutes before Daisy was out and I was so relieved. Daisy arrived looking beautiful because she hadn't been squished on the way out, like the others were. For me, the best thing about all our babies' births was the total relief when it was over and Sally was OK.

Sally wanted a ninth child but I was too worried about the risks after the last pregnancy. When she fell pregnant for the ninth time I called Roger and said, 'She's got me again!' and he laughed. We're his best customers, I think.

I had male postnatal depression after we'd had each child, sulking because I wasn't getting any attention anymore. Sally's attention is divided ten ways now so it feels like there's no attention left for me. I marvel at Sally. She's an unbelievable mum and I really do love being a dad.

My tip to first time dads is to be as caring as you can during the birth. It's scary the first time and she'll need you there. Birth is painful. It really hurts. Hold her hand and encourage her. After the birth, my tip is 'breast is best'. You know why? Because then you don't have to do night feeds!

More kids? NO CHANCE!

CHAPTER 4

UNDERSTANDING LABOUR PAIN

Pain seems to be the most talked about aspect of childbirth. Most women place pain at the top of their list of fears when they are pregnant for the first time and this is based on what they've heard and read, not what they've actually experienced.

According to Sydney obstetrician, Dr John Keogh, pain and perineal tearing top the list of fears for many of the women he cares for.

This was certainly true for me. I had built the pain of childbirth up into the biggest monster fear of all time. As I mentioned, I'd even considered adoption to avoid the pain of childbirth. As a side note, this fear never came from my mother – she always said I slipped out like a wet fish, but then I *was* her fourth child. It was only when I discovered that childbirth didn't have to be hideous that I reframed my thinking and decided it was going to be manageable. I thought that if my mum could handle four drug-free births, then so could I.

Studies[1] on the perception of pain have shown that fearing or anticipating it (or catastrophising pain, as the study says) will actually decrease pain tolerance. This means that your job in the lead up to the birth is to assure your partner that she can handle it and that you'll be there to help her.

Avoid horror stories about the pain of childbirth (tell those who are spouting off about it in front of a pregnant woman that they're not helping her prepare for her birth by making her fearful) and focus on positive pain management rather than treating it as something insurmountable.

Some childbirth educators avoid using the word pain with the couples they work with. In the context of this book, I'm going to call it pain. Some also refer to contractions as waves or surges. I'm going to call them contractions. I call a spade a shovel and I promised I would give it to you straight. It's also in keeping with the lingo used in the usual hospital antenatal classes.

Childbirth *is* painful, but there's an enormous amount that you, the expectant father, can do to help reduce the pain for your partner.

For me, the pain of giving birth was more manageable than I had anticipated. Don't get me wrong – it is full on and ramps up as the labour progresses. But I coped and my husband really made a difference when it came to helping me manage the pain. To be honest, the exhaustion of a long labour bothered me more than the pain.

Here's my analogy for describing the pain of childbirth to a bloke who'll never feel it as long as he lives. The pain of birth is not a destructive, bone crunching or dentist drilling kind of pain. I broke my leg really badly when I was young and reckless and rode a motorcycle. That was a very different kind of pain and much harder to handle than childbirth pain.

Book yourself in for a Chinese massage and ask the guy to go hard on you. That is similar to the kind of pain a woman experiences during a contraction – it is sharp, you want it to stop but you grit your teeth and bear it because you know it won't last forever. It's a muscular kind of pain, like a very powerful stitch or cramp. Now book yourself in for a really hard Chinese massage that goes for say, 12 to 18 hours. You get my drift. You can handle intense pain for a short period of time, but when it goes for hours, you start to lose your sense of humour.

Don't worry about pain thresholds. Lots of women tell me that they have a low pain threshold and this is what scares them most. A research paper on pain[2] suggests that women all have the same pain threshold as such – although there is some research[3] that indicates that redheads have more pain receptors than blondes and brunettes and require more

My wife's worst fear is perineal tearing. What can I do to help prevent it?

The perineum is the tissue between the vagina and the anus. The baby's head stretches this area in a big way. Perineal massage can certainly help prepare the area for the stretch to come and expectant fathers can help with this in the weeks before the birth. 'Using coconut oil or almond oil, men can massage their partner's perineum to help stretch the area,' says midwife Akal Khalsa. 'Massage the area for a few minutes, allowing your partner time to relax and become comfortable with the sensation,' she says, 'then insert two fingers along the back of the vaginal wall, applying firm, consistent, parallel pressure on the perineum and keeping your fingers straight.'

When your partner says she feels a burning sensation, hold the pressure and let her breathe deeply and relax into it. The burning feeling will subside and then you can gently stretch a little more before releasing the pressure. Repeat this two more times. 'Couples can continue to do this each day until it is difficult to cause the burning sensation,' says Akal. 'When this happens, use three fingers and continue in the same way until it is again difficult to cause a burning sensation. Then increase to four fingers. You will both be aware of the increased stretch to the perineum. When you reach a point of maximum stretch, do this every other day to maintain it.'

The position a woman gives birth in is also important in terms of avoiding a tear. Pushing the baby out on all fours or lying on her side with one leg held up takes the weight of the baby off the perineum.

anaesthetic. Apart from redheads, the difference in how women perceive pain is how we are taught to express pain and deal with it socially rather than a genetic predisposition to feeling pain.

Women have a much higher pain tolerance when they are pregnant and in labour: women are built to birth. It's your job to reassure her that she can handle it.

Two basics to aim for

For the most comfortable labour for your partner, you are aiming for two things: a spontaneous labour and a baby in the anterior position.

When it comes to induction, nobody seems to mention that it is much more painful than a spontaneous labour. A drug-induced labour typically produces artificially severe pain with triple peaks on contractions and little rest in between, while a spontaneous labour is generally much more gentle, ramping up gradually. The body's natural pain management hormones are designed to handle a natural labour but they are not equipped to manage one that's drug-induced.

If you are approaching, or have passed your baby's due date, caregivers in a hospital environment will start talking about induction. Some will book your partner in for an induction on the seventh day after the baby's due date, unless you ask for more time. When your partner is feeling heavy and tired and is totally over this pregnancy and the waiting game, the promise of an induction 'and you can have this baby tomorrow' sounds inviting. Weigh up the pros and cons before you settle for an induction that is not medically necessary.

A procedure called sweeping the membranes is a technique that can induce labour without using drugs so this is something to ask your caregiver about if they start talking about induction.

'Couples should be aware that medical induction increases the chance of an epidural and a Caesarean as well as contributing to a higher rate of babies who are admitted to intensive care,' says Associate Professor of Midwifery, Hannah Dahlen. 'Medical induction is not a walk in the park and should not be entered into lightly, just for the sake, for example, of not missing the Grand Final!'

So, what can a man do to avoid a medical induction for his partner?

Is it safe for the baby to go past its due date?

The EDD or estimated due date is just a general indication of when your baby might be due. Only about 3% of babies arrive on their actual due date. Even if you are certain of the exact moment in time that your baby was conceived, you can't be sure of the exact date of arrival. Some babies just take longer to cook than others. Babies are usually considered full term from 37 weeks onwards and are regularly allowed to go up to two weeks past the estimated due date. The main concerns with going overdue are whether the placenta is past its use-by date and therefore no longer sustaining your baby sufficiently, whether there is enough volume of amniotic fluid in the womb to keep the baby healthy and if the baby's size is becoming too large to deliver vaginally. Your caregivers will discuss these issues with you and will keep a close eye on the baby once your partner is overdue. Remember that an induced labour is generally more painful than a spontaneous labour so try to avoid an induction unless it is medically necessary.

There are a number of natural induction techniques that you can try at home but the ones that most couples enjoy amount to a recipe for a great date night: a long walk on the beach, a hot curry and good sex. Most men have no problem with this recommendation for natural induction and some like to put this into practice as soon as possible!

A long walk on the beach lets your partner's hips sway from side to side and lets gravity bring the baby down further into the pelvis. A hot curry is supposed to stimulate digestion. It is also reported to irritate the bowel, which is right next to the uterus. This irritation can jump start the uterus into action.

The last activity to finish off a great Saturday night would be sex.

'There is some evidence that sex works to initiate spontaneous labour, especially in women having their second and subsequent babies,' says Hannah Dahlen. According to Hannah, sex has a three-way action: semen contains prostaglandins which ripen the cervix, an orgasm produces oxytocin, the hormone of love, which also drives labour, and the mechanical impact of sex can motivate labour.

Nipple stimulation also produces oxytocin in your partner's system and most men quite enjoy this task as well. About a minute of nipple stimulation every five minutes simulates the timing of contractions but it needs to be warm and sexy, not a mechanical 'let's try to start labour by turning the key' stimulation.

Run a warm bath, get in there with your partner and see if you can stimulate her nipples to trigger the hormone of love to kickstart labour. These are the last opportunities you have to spend this kind of time together for a while, so make the most of it.

You can also use acupressure to work with the body's pressure points to trigger labour, according to Chinese herbalist and acupuncturist, Naomi Abeshouse. 'Acupressure is a safe and effective, non-invasive way to promote labour and an efficient birth,' says Naomi.

These techniques should not be used before the 38 week mark and each point should be held for about two minutes. Use your knuckles, thumbs, elbows, a tennis ball, dolphin-shaped massage tool, wooden spoon – anything you need to use to apply consistent pressure to the three acupressure points described in the box on the following page.

Positioning of your baby is also important and you want to have your baby in an anterior position for the most comfortable and swift journey through the birth canal. This means that the baby is head down, facing towards your partner's spine, which is much more comfortable for her. A posterior position is the other way around, with the baby's back towards your partner's spine. This causes additional backache, and for some women, no rest from the pain between contractions. Posterior presentations are generally slower and more painful than anterior.

What can you possibly do to influence the position of your baby?

Acupressure points for natural induction of labour

- *SP6 helps to ripen the cervix. This point is on the inside of the lower leg, four of the labouring woman's finger-widths up from the bone that protrudes from the inside of the ankle. This area will often be tender and the point can be found when you slide your finger off the edge of the tibia bone, towards the inside of the leg. This point can be given pressure once or twice a day on each leg.*

- *GB21 helps your baby descend and engage for women birthing for the first time. This point is at the base of her neck and can be given pressure as part of a good, firm shoulder massage, at least three times a week.*

- *BL31 and BL32 support an efficient birth, help the cervix dilate and can help with pain relief during prelabour. These acupressure points lie midway between the dimples above the buttocks and the lumbar spine. If you can't see the dimples clearly, this point is roughly one of your partner's index finger-lengths above the top of the buttock crease and about one thumb-width either side of the spine. When you place your finger on this point you can feel the small depression of the sacral foramen, where the point lies. You can work these points at least three times a week. Sit your partner in a chair with her back towards you and her upper body resting on the back of the chair and give her a good lower back rub with extra emphasis on these pressure points.*

To see online video demonstrations of these acupressure points, search YouTube by the pressure point names referred to above.

There are two common opinions on this.

According to birth consultant Denise Love, to encourage your baby to be in an anterior position your partner needs to spend as much time as possible during her third trimester on all fours with her pelvis tipped forward. Denise recommends having a beanbag so that your partner can flop forward to watch TV while you give her a back rub. And none of this 'my arms are tired' excuse. Your partner needs a one-hour back and shoulder rub every night of her last trimester.

Denise recommends that women in their last trimester lie on their left side to prevent a posterior birth and, 'A woman should avoid reclining back in a comfy couch at home or in a chair at work. She should sit on the edge of her seat with her pelvis tipped forward as much as possible as this encourages the baby to be in the anterior position,' says Denise.

'In my 35-year career of helping women birth their babies, including work in countries like Thailand, Cambodia and Nepal, I've never seen nearly as many posterior presentations as I have in Australia,' she says. 'Women in Australia don't get down on their hands and knees to clean their homes anymore. They're not the ones scrubbing the floors. Many women in Australia recline back in a chair at work and then lie on the couch at home watching DVDs.'

Women in countries like Cambodia, where Denise and her husband Gary have set up a birth centre, spend their time squatting or on their knees as they work in the fields throughout their pregnancies.

However, a randomised controlled trial[4] published in 2004 concluded that time spent on all fours together with pelvic rocking from 37 weeks onwards had no influence on preventing persistent posterior positioning.

Obstetrician Dr John Keogh, one of the authors of the published paper on this trial, says that only 3% of women actually deliver their babies in a posterior position. About 20% of women have a posterior presentation during labour and most of those turn during labour to be delivered in the more comfortable anterior presentation.

According to Dr Keogh, the three most important factors to influence the baby's position during labour are efficient contractions, adequate pain relief and remaining mobile as long as the woman can.

'When a woman is in a lot of pain, she's very tense. If she can be given adequate pain relief, she will be able to relax, let go and allow more room in the pelvis for her baby to turn.'

Depending on your preferences, you may like to consider natural attempts to encourage your baby to be in the anterior position before labour commences, knowing that once your partner is in labour, you have the help of your caregivers to encourage your baby to turn.

Know your hormones

It's important to understand some of the hormones in your partner's body in order to support her effectively. She is a cocktail of hormones when she's pregnant, in labour and postpartum, but there are only three you need to know and understand to support her effectively in labour.

Endorphins are the body's natural painkillers. They are the buzz you get during and after exercise, excitement and orgasm: it's all very sexy, this childbirth caper. Endorphins act like opiates in their ability to produce analgesia and a feeling of wellbeing. They are said to be 300 times more powerful than morphine. Morphine is a fabulous painkiller! It knocks your socks off. I've had my fair share of morphine with all those operations to my leg and I found the claim that endorphins are 300 times more powerful than morphine to be a little hard to believe. However, the power of endorphins was demonstrated very well to me when I gave birth to my first.

The day before our son was born, a midwife had given me an acupuncture treatment to encourage labour to start. She had put a number of needles in a few places and then attached an electronic pulse machine to some of them. This machine had a dial, which went from one to ten. I had to turn the dial to the highest level at which I could tolerate the vibrating discomfort. I could handle five on the dial at the absolute most, at a time when I was not in labour.

I had booked another acupuncture treatment for the next day, but I was already in labour when the midwife arrived, so she used the treatment to kick labour into the established stage. When I was in labour, with my endorphins starting to do their job, I could turn the dial up to ten without even feeling it. I even double-checked that it was actually turned on. This gave me immense confidence in my own body to manage the pain.

To keep endorphins flowing in the body, a woman needs to be in the pain of labour. The natural reaction to the pain is the production of this amazing hormone. She also needs to keep moving gently.

Oxytocin drives contractions and keeps labour going. Nothing is more demoralising than a labour that doesn't keep going. A stop-start labour is exhausting. Your partner needs a good flow of oxytocin to keep contractions coming. This is often referred to as the hormone of love or the cuddle chemical: it makes you feel good and it's released when a woman is in labour, when she breastfeeds and when she has sex.

'When they're with a birthing woman, all the care providers release oxytocin in their own systems,' says Hannah Dahlen. 'That's why midwives are addicted to birth. You can *feel* the love in the room.'

To keep oxytocin flowing, a woman needs to stay upright. This helps to bring the baby down, putting pressure on the cervix, which stimulates oxytocin production.

Many women make the mistake of getting into the bath and lying on their back for a nice soak early in labour. They should be upright to keep the labour cranking.

Our mothers' generation was told to lie on a bed while in labour and to stay still and quiet, so they did it much tougher than women birthing today who are generally encouraged to move around and stay upright in order to help those key hormones work their magic.

Adrenalin blocks endorphins and oxytocin. If this is the only thing you remember from this book, your job is to make sure your partner has as little adrenalin in her system as possible. This hormone is produced by all the negative feelings such as embarrassment, irritation, frustration, fear, panic and anger.

If you are annoying your partner, if there are four student doctors with clipboards standing at the end of her bed, if the midwife keeps leaving the door open and your partner feels that anyone can hear her labour, if the resident doctor on the ward is a creep, if you smell, if you're having a verbal biffo with the midwife, if your partner is anxious that this labour will never end… any of these things will produce adrenalin and make your partner's labour longer and harder. It sounds overly sensitive, but as I have said, women in labour are.

Adrenalin is designed to stall labour or at least slow it down if there is an immediate danger to the mother. While your partner is not in the kind of danger that your average cave woman faced, she still needs to feel completely safe, protected, supported and loved. This is your job.

So remember: endorphins and oxytocin are your friends. Adrenalin is the enemy.

The most important things to remember about the pain of childbirth and how it works are:

- *Aim for a spontaneous labour with no induction unless medically necessary*
- *Consider natural induction techniques*
- *Aim for a baby in the anterior position*
- *Know your hormones: endorphins nuke the pain, oxytocin drives the labour but adrenalin blocks them both*
- *Do whatever you have to do to make your partner feel safe, protected, supported and loved*

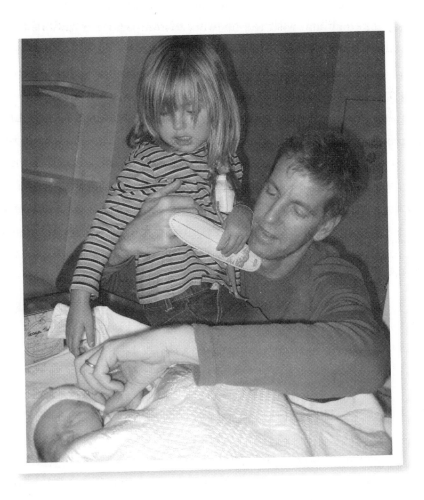

JAMES TOMKINS' STORY

If only you could harness the intensity and endurance of childbirth and put that in a boat – you'd have a winner.

James Tomkins AOM tried his hand at rowing on his second day at Carey Grammar School in Melbourne in 1979. At six foot six, he was well suited to the sport and liked the water. Three decades later, he is a three-time Olympic gold medallist and one of only a few Australian athletes to have competed at six Olympic Games. James has won seven gold medals at the World Championships and is the only rower in history to win titles in every sweep-oared class at this event. His coxless four team earned the legendary nickname, the Oarsome Foursome, after winning gold in the Barcelona Olympics in 1992 and then again at the 1996 Atlanta Olympics. At the Sydney 2000 Olympics, James raced in the coxless pair, winning bronze, and went on to win gold a third time in Athens in 2004. He has an economics and finance degree and has worked in the finance industry through much of his elite sporting career. James and his wife Bridget have three young daughters, including twins. In 2008, James won the Victorian Father's Day Council's Father of the Year Award.

We thought we had miscarried our first daughter, Jessica. She was conceived while we were travelling in America and then a few weeks later, Bridget had all the symptoms of a miscarriage. We're not sure, but we think we actually lost Jess's twin, but we thought that Bridget was no longer pregnant. We went on with our travels and I coached the US rowing team for some of that time. We did some big hikes and went out a lot – not ideal for a pregnancy that we weren't aware of. A little later, when we were in Switzerland, we did a six-hour hike up Mount Pilatus and Bridget was absolutely knackered, which was not like her. And there I was, thinking, 'Come on!'

At sixteen weeks, we found out that Bridget was still pregnant. The doctor in the US said Bridget had a blood clot which made it a very high-risk pregnancy. We sent the reports back to Australia and were told that it was all fine. I think that's the difference between Australia and the US. It was all about the worst-case scenario over there.

Giving birth is a bit like racing. You spend months preparing for it and then you wake up on that morning and it all comes down to this: you can't back out. As a rower, you concentrate on one event each year for the World Championships and only once every four years for the Olympic Games. On the morning of a race, there's this massive sense of dread. On that day, you can't hide from your own performance. I think it's the same for a woman giving birth. She can't back out!

Bridget was amazing the day she gave birth. It was all natural, no drugs except for a bit of gas. The labour was about twelve hours long so I went off and did some training while she was in early labour as I was twiddling my thumbs with nothing to do. The midwives were all fussing around and her contractions were just little fluffy ones at that stage. She was laughing, thinking it was pretty easy, but she wasn't dilating yet.

I think my wife contributed to the Melbourne water shortage because once labour really got going she sat on a Swiss ball in the shower for about six hours with the water running. I tried to give her something to concentrate on other than the pain. I sat on another Swiss ball in my boardies doing a bit of core stability work in the shower. I had my stopwatch and was checking her heart rate. I think I needed to check my own! And there was a bit of barracking to cheer her on.

I suppose I approached the birth like an athlete. You have to sequence through the event in a structured way. A race only lasts for about six minutes but you have to have a strategy. Do it well and the outcome will be good. If only you could harness the intensity and endurance of childbirth and put that in a boat – you'd have a winner. Bridget's endurance, her ability to hang in there just blew me away.

When Jess was born, it was amazing. I stayed up the bowler's end and didn't venture down to the batter's end. It's totally different compared to winning an Olympic medal. That's all about you. This time I was more concerned about my wife. It looked like a shotgun murder in that room – the mess! I cut the cord, which was a bit gristly.

When we took our baby home we thought, 'Now what do we do?' It was easy in the hospital with help from the midwives, but when you get home, you're on your own for the rest of your life. On the very first night at home we put Jess in a little alcove just outside our room. That lasted about two hours! She was too noisy so we put her down the hall.

Sport is structured and disciplined. We approached our newborn baby in the same way with a routine and a bit of self-discipline, which made things easier down the track. We tried to roll with the punches and work it out as we went and Jess is a delightful, gorgeous child.

After Athens it was time to think about another baby. With the first pregnancy, Bridget had the timing of her cycle all wrong. Only when she'd read the 'instruction manual', did we get the timing right and she fell pregnant. In fact, the second time, we only had to think about it and she was pregnant.

It was a massive shock to find out that we were having twins. The ultrasound doctor was checking everything: 'Head, spine, heart; head, spine, heart.' We said, 'What?' and he said, 'I take it no one's told you that you're having twins?' I was numb. Holy hell. We didn't know anyone who had twins back then. Now they seem like a dime a dozen.

Our girls are fraternal twins and I thought I was pretty clever to be able to sire two kids in one go. I have good swimmers – as you'd expect. My wife's had three kids with only one and half pregnancies.

Bridget's belly was huge with the twins. She's skinny but I thought her stomach was going to pop!

We had a scheduled Caesarean, which was a bit stressful. I was trying to be light-hearted and was all gowned up like the doctor, pretending to take her pulse. In the end the midwives asked me to move some furniture in another part of the hospital, just to get rid of me. Maybe I was getting a little over-excited.

The epidural didn't work right away and this made Bridget anxious. I stayed up the bowler's end again. Once they got in there, it was like rustling around to find a screwdriver at the bottom of a tool chest. They had to dig around and then the first baby was out.

We had found out the gender earlier because we didn't want to have to think of four names. Holly was first and then Georgia. They looked beautiful. Bridget held them on her chest while they stitched her up.

When we arrived home from the hospital with the twins, the snoozers from ASADA [*Australian Sports Anti-Doping Authority*] were standing on our doorstep saying I had been selected for a random drug test. Bridget wasn't impressed.

Having twins was full on but it's not double the work. Bridget breastfed using a big feeding cushion with a baby under each arm like a scrum. She thought it was great to have all the night-time sport to watch: the Ashes, Tour de France, Wimbledon, Masters Golf.

We took the government baby bonus and spent it on a night nurse who came and stayed with us three nights a week for about ten weeks. Bridget would get up at night to feed the girls and then the nurse would settle them and put them back to bed. This worked brilliantly. It was the best dough we ever spent.

Three and a half was the perfect age for Jess to have her sisters arrive. She was gentle with them and made them laugh. The three of them have distinct personalities. Holly came out squawking and hasn't changed since. Georgia needed a little oxygen when she was born and is the more quiet, laid back character.

Being a father has helped me put sport into perspective. It made me see that rowing is just sitting in a boat and rowing on a lake or a river. It's a pretty simple thing to do.

In elite sport, it is all about you, with your partner supporting you. You have a physiologist, physiotherapist, nutritionist, boat builder, weight trainer – an entire team. You have to be disciplined and selfish. When it comes to being a father, it's not all about you anymore. I needed to fend for my wife to make sure she wasn't exhausted. We didn't pander to the child's every whim but took a balanced approach to meeting the baby's needs and Bridget's needs for rest. I tried to be attuned to what Bridget needed but it was always a bit of a mystery.

Of the six guys that I rowed with in the coxless four, there are eleven kids between us and nine of them are girls. I'm told this has something to do with testosterone. There's plenty of that in sport!

CHAPTER 5

PRACTICAL IDEAS FOR PAIN MANAGEMENT

You don't need to be a helpless onlooker when it comes to the birth of your baby and this is no spectator sport. One of the reasons why I created the Beer + Bubs workshops was that I had so often heard men say how helpless they'd felt at the births of their babies. They said they felt useless and disempowered. They hated watching their partner suffer and felt that they couldn't save her from what she was going through. For many men, their most profound memory of the birth of their baby was their partner pleading with them to put her out of her misery. There was nothing they felt that they could DO to help her through the pain and the helplessness was horrid.

That is not the case at all if you know what you're doing. While you can't *save* your partner from what she is going through, you can certainly help with her pain management in a hands-on way. You should be almost as exhausted as the birthing mother by the time your baby is born because you've been so involved. There's a lot to do…

Some of you may have done hypnosis-style classes and while they are an excellent birth preparation, having some active birth techniques on your list is important for the later stages of labour. I am yet to support a woman who, birthing for the first time, has used only hypnosis and breathing techniques for her entire labour and birth. There's no reason why you can't combine hypnosis techniques with being up and active.

I believe that when you are supporting a woman through childbirth, you need to go in with an arsenal of weapons to use against the pain.

This can include everything from heat packs at home to an epidural in hospital and you'll have numerous things you can try before you get to that epidural.

Even if your partner has no interest in a natural birth, you will still need to help her manage the pain until the drugs take effect.

Engage the senses for an active birth

The idea behind the following pain management techniques is to actively engage several of the senses in order to confuse the nerve pathways of the brain so that there is only so much brain capacity left with which to perceive the pain. Simple but effective. So, let's talk through the senses…

Touch

Heat is said to reduce pain by 40%. Heat packs are great in early labour and I recommend gel packs. This type of heat pack has a disc or button floating around inside which you click. The sudden movement triggers a chemical reaction so that the sodium acetate inside instantly heats up, then stays hot for about an hour.

Many hospitals won't let you use microwave heat packs and the ones they give you in hospitals are hopeless. They don't mould well to the body and they are nowhere near hot enough. Give a woman in labour a luke-warm heat pack and watch how fast she lobs it across the room.

Invest in two or three gel packs and after the birth you can use them for your own aching muscles after a game of footy. The small ones make great hand-warmers when you go fishing. For your partner's pain relief, place one heat pack below her navel and one on her lower back.

The bath is also a great tool for managing pain. I call it 'the big gun'. When a woman says, 'I've had enough, I want an epidural!' I say, 'Let's get in the bath.' Just make sure she's not diving in there too early in the labour and that she stays on all fours or sitting on her heels. Most baths in hospitals take a long time to fill so you'll need to start filling it before she needs it. Usually the hot water tap on full with no cold water is hot but not too hot for your partner. She will want it as hot as possible but just be careful that you don't burn her. The midwives should keep an eye on the temperature of the water and won't let you run it too hot.

The shower is excellent for pain management too and there are usually two removable showerheads available in birthing suites that have a shower. Turn the taps off (or in the bath, turn the spa pump off) between contractions so that the heat hits her lower back for the best effect during each contraction.

Massage will keep you very busy. I believe that men were made with muscles to massage women in labour! She needs strong, deep U-shaped massage at the base of her spine. Some women don't like to be touched when they are in labour, but it is usually the wussy, floppy touch of a tired, distracted man that drives a woman nuts. Women in labour prefer a strong touch. If you pat her gently or tickle her, she *will* hit you.

Use a labour massage oil or contact an aromatherapist to make one up for you that includes the essential oil, clary sage. Clary sage usually smells like wet dog so it is often combined with an essential oil like lavender or sandalwood.

'Sandalwood is very strengthening and brings peace of mind but has a heady scent and a small amount goes a long way,' says Canberra-based childbirth educator and aromatherapist, Vickie Hingston-Jones. 'Any citrus oil blends well with clary sage.'

Essential oil in its natural state is too strong to be used directly on the skin and needs to be blended with a massage base oil. For every single drop of essential oil add 2mls of massage base oil. There are a number of suitable base oils but Vickie recommends sweet almond oil which is light and good for general massage.

'Don't buy cheap oils, they don't work effectively and are false economy,' says Vickie. 'Individual oils can be purchased from health food shops and department stores. If you are unsure, contact an aromatherapist (listed in the yellow pages) who can also make up a blend for you.'

Sound

Encourage vocalisation. They say that an open throat is an open cervix, so encourage your partner to *ahhhhhhh* through contractions with an open throat. The most common reaction to pain is a pained cry, so help your partner to turn that painful sound into an open-throated *ahhhhhhh* sound. She is using her larynx, she's hearing her own sounds and she's engaging another sense.

Music is great to use during childbirth but make sure it's music without lyrics so as not to engage the language centres of the brain. Make sure it's music that *she* likes. Whatever you put on first will probably be what you will listen to for the rest of the labour so my advice is not to put on Enya first! It'll drive you insane after several hours.

My suggestion is to put together about a ten hour playlist of instrumental classical or ambient music on an MP3 player and take your own MP3 speakers with you. Hit repeat and you've got enough music to last you a long time before you notice that you've heard anything three times. If you use an iPhone as your MP3 player, set it to airplane mode so that you don't receive calls or texts.

I've noticed that the most common thing that men forget to take to the birth is music. If this happens, just find a classical radio station. Most hospitals have a portable stereo provided in the birth suites.

Smell

Aromatherapy oils are used by many doulas and midwives to engage the sense of smell in childbirth. According to Vickie Hingston-Jones, correctly used aromatherapy oils have specific medicinal qualities that can reduce stress and discomfort.

'When an essential oil is inhaled, the molecules enter the nasal cavity and stimulate the limbic system in the brain,' says Vickie. 'This is the region of the brain that influences emotions and memories and is directly linked to the adrenal and pituitary glands and the hypothalamus. These are the parts of the body that regulate heart rate, blood pressure, stress, hormone balance and breathing. The effects of essential oils can immediately bring about both emotional and physiological balance.'

Vickie stresses that it is very important to use only natural essential oils made from plants and flowers. Synthetic oils, often labelled as fragrant oils, do not contain any therapeutic qualities, can cause headaches and nausea and have none of the benefits that natural plant oils provide.

To use aromatherapy in your partner's pain management routine, place a few drops of neat essential oil on a washer or tissue and then let your partner inhale the smell right before a contraction. The smell will flood the senses and give her brain something else to perceive, other than the pain. Another sense is engaged and the pain has less of the brain's attention.

Vicky suggests lime oil (citrus aurantifolia) for pain management as it is also a restorative tonic. 'Use lime oil to energise a tired mind and beat fatigue and anxiety. Lime is very good for both parents, especially when labour has been going for a long time,' says Vickie. 'Other citrus oils like mandarin and grapefruit are also good.'

Peppermint oil (menthe piperita) is used for reducing anxiety, pain, nausea and vomiting during labour. 'Peppermint is an excellent wake-up oil when energy is at its lowest, especially during the peak of labour,' says Vickie.

You can also use these oils in an oil burner, with many hospitals providing electric burners in their birth suites.

Take care with all essential oils as they are highly concentrated and should not come in contact with your new baby. Wash your hands well after using them.

Sight

A visual focus can be very helpful but I have to admit, this is one of the last tricks I pull out of my doula bag. I usually try other more active techniques first. I have a box of black and white images and I choose one to put in front of the woman so that she can concentrate on it during contractions. Women usually want to keep the image as a memento.

You could give your partner something to focus on that reminds her that she's having a baby. It's easy to forget this detail when you're in the throes of labour. A little size 0000 singlet or a bonnet that you have packed for your baby will give her something to focus on visually and will also bring her mental focus back to the baby she is birthing.

Taste

This is the last of the senses that is engaged during labour and is least useful in pain management. All the breathing that your partner will be doing will make her mouth taste awful so some barley sugar or mints will help clear her tongue and will also give her one more sensory focus.

Movement

Movement is very important to keep endorphins working effectively but remember to conserve energy; you might be at this for a couple of days. Birth balls are available in most hospitals and these are great because she can sit on the birth ball and rock from side to side so that she's not on her feet for most of the labour. She can lean her upper body on the bed while she rocks on the birth ball.

Establish a pain management routine

Use these techniques to establish a pain management routine that you use with your partner. If something works, she won't want to change it, so you may be doing the same thing for hours and hours. If the worst thing that happens during this birth is that you are bored to snores, you're doing OK. If she hates something that you introduce, don't worry, just move on. If she likes something, stick with it.

When I was in established labour, I inhaled lime oil on a wash cloth, bounced on a birth ball, *ahhhh*-ed the house down, stared at a visual focus on our bedroom wall and held a heat pack below my belly, while Bruce massaged my lower back furiously. It was quite a song and dance but it managed the pain extremely well and had Bruce very involved in a hands-on and helpful way. He really felt that he was part of the team, getting me through each contraction. I got all the way to seven or eight centimetres dilated before I started to lose my sense of humour. All this sensory activity busied the brain and left little mental capacity for the pain.

Pharmacological pain relief

You may also be called on to help your partner when it comes to the use of drugs for pain relief. In Australian hospitals, there are a number of options to consider.

The least invasive drug on offer is gas. This comes out of a pipe in the wall in the birth suite and is nitrous oxide (laughing gas) mixed with oxygen. Your partner must hold the mouth-piece herself because it is self dosing. Once she has had enough she will go floppy and won't be able to hold it any longer. If you're holding it for her she'll have too much and it might make her sick.

The good thing about gas is that it is out of her system quickly, so if she hates it you can stop using it and the effects will wear off promptly. Some women say the sound of the ball in the mouthpiece is the most effective part of the gas. Others say it doesn't necessarily reduce the pain, it just calms them down so that the pain bothers them a lot less.

Did I mention that this is not a very glamorous job? Some women vomit throughout labour, in which case you will be the Vomit Bucket Man. Gas can make some women throw up but that is usually short-lived since the gas leaves the system quickly.

There is also pethidine on offer (or morphine, depending on which one your caregiver is more accustomed to administering) but this comes in a four-hour dose as a jab in the thigh. If she doesn't like it, she's stuck feeling like a space cadet for four hours. My colleague Jane says that she hated pethidine. It made her very sleepy and she dozed off between contractions which meant she had no mental break from the pain. Each contraction would hit and wake her up suddenly. Pethidine also made her puke for hours and she felt completely out of control.

Women who are labouring with a baby in the posterior position often have significant back pain. In this situation, some obstetricians and midwives offer sterile water injections. This is a very effective method of pain relief, triggering pain receptors in the skin to reorder the brain's pain hierarchy. This effectively gives external pain receptors priority over internal receptors, cutting the signal between the internal back pain and the brain.

'A series of four 1ml injections of sterile water into the skin across a woman's back will give her about an hour and half of relief from severe back pain associated with the later stages of posterior labour,' says obstetrician Dr John Keogh. 'It stings like a wasp for about 30 seconds initially but it is the sting that triggers the response.'

If your partner opts for this method, it's important that you don't rub or massage the injection sites or the treatment will lose its effectiveness.

The next option for pain relief is an epidural. I could probably write a whole book on just the pros and cons of epidurals. As mentioned previously, it can be a touchy subject.

Some believe that epidurals are to be avoided because they begin the slippery slope into lots of other medical interventions. The risks involved with epidurals are rare but serious: spinal damage, infections, heart attack and even death. These will be explained to you by the anaesthetist before the epidural is applied. However, your partner will be in immense pain by then and not really able to make an informed decision, so it's best to discuss the risks you are taking with an epidural well before the birth and decide how you both feel about this pain relief option.

I have been at births when an epidural was the best option for that baby to be delivered vaginally rather than surgically, giving the woman a chance to rest and relax while her cervix dilated so that she had the energy to push her baby out when the time came. However, I have also seen an epidural go in when the woman was nine centimetres dilated and then it's really unnecessary.

In a normal vaginal birth, an epidural is a choice, not a medical necessity.

The obvious benefit of an epidural is total pain relief when the drug works effectively. However, women who have an epidural are more likely to have an instrumental delivery[5] (forceps or vacuum) and many women find the numbness difficult to 'push through' when it comes time to push their baby out. The dose can be turned down so that a woman has more sensation in the pushing stage but this leaves her on her back, on the bed, attached to a monitor, drips and a catheter (to drain the bladder) and with few natural resources to manage the pain she finds herself in again.

Talk to your caregivers and discuss epidurals with your partner well before the birth. In my experience, if a woman doesn't have a really good reason *not* to have an epidural, she will opt for one. That good reason might be fear of other interventions or fear of needles, or perhaps she really wants to have a drug free labour and have her senses alive when she gives birth. She just needs to have a good reason that she's committed to if she wants to avoid an epidural.

Expectant fathers often ask me how to handle the situation if their partner doesn't want an epidural, but in the throes of labour starts begging for one. Just about every woman I have ever supported has asked for an epidural during labour – even the ones with the most natural of birth plans. So it's natural for her to ask.

'Most women beg for an epidural at about seven centimetres, even if they're dead against it,' says Denise Love who has supported over 4000 couples in her career as a doula. 'Your job is to get them through it, one contraction at a time.'

Denise says that she has often observed an interesting behaviour pattern in women who are losing the plot and begging for pain relief. 'A woman can be screaming and begging for an epidural, climbing the walls in agony, literally throwing herself around the room. When it comes to letting the anaesthetist put a needle into her spine, and I look her in the eyes and say, "You need to stay perfectly still or you'll never walk again," she will somehow be able to regulate her breathing and stay perfectly still, as if in an hypnotic trance. This can take up to twenty minutes. To me this shows that she just needs a reason to manage with her own resources and hold it together and she can do it.'

If your partner really, truly doesn't want an epidural and would like to avoid drugs in labour, the best thing you can do is distract her. Just keep her focused on the next contraction and then the one after that. If she's begging for an epidural, then her natural pain management techniques aren't working for her, so change what you are doing. Get her into the bath, work harder at massaging her back and introduce some other sensory stimulation. Perhaps you could suggest she try some gas.

If, on the other hand, she has always been open to having an epidural if she felt she needed it, then it's time to call the midwife and get an anaesthetist in there quick smart. If she's decided she wants an epidural, don't stand in her way. She'll hate you for it!

Dr John Keogh says, 'I have heard men say to their wives, who are in enormous pain and begging for an epidural, "No, no. You don't need pain relief!" However, the only person who knows how much pain she is in is the woman in labour. Sometimes people make a plan before labour not to have a particular sort of pain relief, but in labour the plan may need to change. If the woman changes her mind about something, her husband needs to avoid rigidly trying to keep her on track. It's a hard path to walk.'

Warning to all men: women fall in love with their anaesthetists. He arrives like a knight in shining armour with a trolley of goodies and the skills and experience to apply a drug to the spine that completely takes the pain away. Most women hold a special place in their heart for the person who did that for them!

If your partner opts for an epidural, you need to help her stay very still for the metal shaft to be inserted into her spine. She'll be asked either to lie on her side, curled up in a ball, or to sit on the bed and curl over to open up the vertebrae for the needle to go into the spinal canal.

Insist that this is done *only* between contractions. I have seen an anaesthetist try to push the epidural needle in during a contraction when a woman can't possibly keep absolutely still.

If you are squeamish, don't watch it going in as it takes a bit of force to puncture the epidural space. It's not a needle really, but a metal shaft that is inserted after a local anaesthetic numbs the area, then a fine catheter is fed through the shaft. The shaft is then removed, leaving the catheter in position, which is taped in place.

It takes about half an hour before the drug is working properly so you'll still have to help her with her pain management until then but she'll be limited to lying on the bed and various monitoring devices will be attached to her belly.

You may have heard of a walking epidural, which is designed to give a woman pain relief so that she can still walk around. However, the epidural comes with a drip connected to a canula in your partner's arm, a catheter to drain her bladder, with a bag for collecting the urine, as well as constant foetal monitoring, which has her connected to another device by cables, which are connected to two large elastic straps across your partner's belly.

'Walking epidurals are a bit of myth,' says Hannah Dahlen. 'The pain relief is often not that effective and by the time you have all the hardware connected, she's not walking anywhere! Her movement is limited by all that equipment. Furthermore, very few anaesthetists offer this method.'

Some women feel a sense of failure for opting for an epidural, especially if they had hoped to avoid one, so stay positive and remind her that she'll be giving birth soon. Some women don't have any expectations at all in terms of avoiding pharmacological pain relief. You'll know where your partner stands and how you can support her best at this stage of the game.

If you're past the due date, your partner could go into labour at any minute and you have only just picked up this book, these are the points to remember:

- *Refer to the pain management arsenal list below*
- *Get involved! This is a hands-on job*
- *Develop a pain management routine*
- *Engage the senses*
- *Let your partner hold the mouth piece for the gas herself*
- *Help her stay very still for the needle if she has an epidural*

Your pain management arsenal:

- *Heat packs*
- *Massage*
- *Vocalisation*
- *Music*
- *Aromatherapy oils*
- *Movement*
- *Visual focus*
- *Bath or shower*
- *Gas*
- *Sterile water injections*
- *Pethidine or morphine*
- *Epidural*

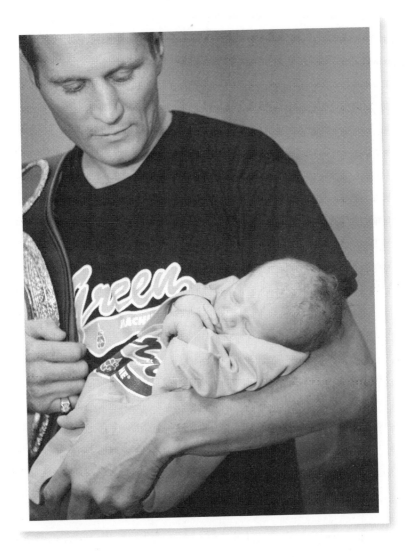

Photo Tony McDonough, The Sunday Times

DANNY GREEN'S STORY

I would rather be put in the ring with Mike Tyson, Evander Holyfield and George Foreman, all at once, than have to go through childbirth.

Boxer Danny Green began his amateur career at the age of 18 after boxing in the back shed in suburban Perth as a kid. He KOed his first amateur opponent in his first match and has been knocking out opponents ever since, winning 29 professional bouts out of 32. Danny won an Institute of Sport scholarship to train for the Commonwealth Games and the 2000 Sydney Olympics, after which he launched his professional boxing career. He went on to win three world titles in the super middleweight, light heavyweight and cruiser weight divisions. Danny is gifted with what he calls 'sleeping pills' in both hands, a resilience to pain that has seen him crowned world champion in this most brutal of sports. With all this under his belt, Danny still believes that the births of his two children rate as the greatest personal achievements of his life. He keeps winning fights and in between, reports to his kids' school for canteen duty.

My daughter Chloe was born in 2002, just four days before my eighth professional fight. My wife Nina was scheduled for an induction the night before the fight, but I said, 'Doc, can I have a quick word with you? This fight is a big deal and I don't want to miss the birth of my child. Can we have it out sooner?' I had also done my research and I knew that she was already well overdue and I didn't want to leave it too late for the baby's sake either.

'No problem, Mr Green,' says the doctor and Nina was induced four days before the fight.

We didn't go to one prenatal class or read one book to prepare for childbirth, so neither of us had any idea of what to expect. I guess we were a bit unorthodox in that sense. We figured that people give birth all over the world every day without attending antenatal classes and even without doctors, so we thought we'd be fine.

When it came down to it, I found the birth of our first child confronting and intimidating, but exciting at the same time. It was nature in its most raw state.

Nina found walking was the best thing to do during contractions, so I walked with her, holding her hand. Between contractions I shadow boxed around the room. The next contraction would come and I'd grab her and rub her lower back, then get back to my shadow boxing once the contraction had passed. The boxing occupied me and helped me keep prepared for the fight at the same time.

'You are a dickhead!' Nina said to me at one point.

I tried to make Nina laugh, which I think helped to kill any fear she had but the labour was about five hours long and she'd had enough of me by the end. She'd probably say I was a half-wit, but that it was good having me there all the same.

To be honest, if I were to watch another lady give birth, I think it would be hideous, horrendous! But because it was my wife and my child, it was beautiful.

The feeling when Chloe was born was indescribable. I looked her in the eyes and I was mesmerised. Words really don't do the feeling any justice. It was incredible. I used to tell my mates, 'Do not miss the birth. It's the best thing you'll ever do.'

Four days later, I won the fight against Iobe Ledua in the second round. I just wanted it over and done with so that I could go home and see Chloe again. Afterwards the media were asking me all the usual post-fight questions, but I just wanted to get away and see my beautiful baby daughter.

Winning three world titles doesn't compare with creating a beautiful human being. Nina and I created our babies and they're flesh and blood. A successful boxing career doesn't even come close to that.

Archie's birth was a lot longer and harder. Nina had a fever during the 18-hour labour and she shook uncontrollably. We held hands and she just about crushed mine. Luckily I have good tolerance to pain, especially in my hands.

Archie was due on the day that I was fighting Stipe Drews for the world title. Nina had contractions that morning and I'm praying, 'Please God, not today!' Nina held on and Archie was born six days later.

A new baby and a world title in one week are hard to top.

I had a strong gut feeling about the gender of both of our babies. We didn't find out whether they were going to be a girl or boy before they were born, but I just had this strong gut feeling that didn't waver throughout each pregnancy.

I knew that Archie was going to be a boy. I had a bet with the doctor who said, 'You know, most athletes have girls,' and I said, 'I'm telling you now, this baby is a boy!' and he says, 'No way, Mr Green!' In those last chaotic moments before Archie was born by forceps delivery, I bet my house on it! The midwife said, 'Can you please be quiet, you two?'

Archie was born and I was right! I said, 'He's got a ball bag, Doc!' I was so thrilled to have a son – and win the bet.

Nina wasn't too keen on the name Archie. I helped cut the cord and then took him over to the table where the midwife put his hospital name bands on his little wrists. She asked me what his name was and I said, 'Archie Malcolm Green!' then I took him back over to Nina and she was too dazed to care.

I wrote a poem which is in my autobiography [*Closed Fists, Open Heart*, published in 2008 by ABC Books]. It's called Heartwarmers and expresses just how much I love Chloe and Archie and how I'm looking forward to our future as a family.

To be honest, it still freaks me out that a baby can grow inside a human being in the first place, but then for it to come out and breathe on its own is wild!

I would rather be put in the ring with Mike Tyson, Evander Holyfield and George Foreman all at once than have to go through childbirth, for sure. Dealing with pain in boxing is a mental thing. I just decide to shut it out and deal with it later, after the fight or after training. Childbirth goes on for such a long time though. It's so heavy. I'm in awe of what women can do and how much pain they can handle. I have such respect for Nina and for women in general. A female is a very durable, tough human creature.

I'm a pretty hands-on dad. I travel a lot and train a lot, but when I'm home, I'm home and I'm all theirs.

I did canteen duty yesterday and I was fleeced for ten bucks! Some kid says to me, 'What can I get for twenty cents, Mr Green?' and I said, 'Nothin' mate!' Then I put down ten bucks and said, 'Order whatever you like, son.' He thought all his Christmases had come at once.

When Chloe was about four months old, we couldn't get a babysitter for one of my fights and she came along and slept in the pram. The noise of that crowd could have woken up people in Siberia but she slept right through it. She's carried the flag out for me at the start of a fight once but she hasn't seen me fight.

I'm not a violent person outside the ring but once the bell goes, my job is to win. If someone tried to hurt my family I think I would mutate! I tell the kids that what I do is just sport and people pay to watch the sport. People get hurt playing other sports like rugby league as well. Boxing is a game. It's a tough game but that's all it is.

CHAPTER 6

SUPPORTING YOUR PARTNER THROUGH LOSS

This book doesn't seek to focus on what can go wrong, as the vast majority of pregnancies in Australia are uncomplicated and healthy. However, stillbirth is a terrible loss that requires a father-to-be to support his partner in the same practical ways as if she were giving birth to a healthy baby, but with an aftermath of utter grief rather than joy.

About 99.5% of births in Australia and New Zealand are live births, which means about 1 in every 200 babies is stillborn[1]. Of these, almost a third remain unexplained.

A baby born with no signs of life is a stillbirth. If the birth occurs before 20 weeks gestation it is classified as a miscarriage. Both are heartbreaking but for stillborn babies there is a legal requirement for the birth and death of the child to be registered.

In her book *Pregnancy Loss: Surviving Miscarriage and Stillbirth* journalist Zoe Taylor tackles the subject of pregnancy loss with bravery and sensitivity, having experienced her own repeated pregnancy losses.

'Often, the mother of a stillborn baby knows that she is going to deliver a baby who is no longer alive,' says Zoe. 'Sometimes that is discovered after the waters break and/or premature labour begins. A common scenario, however, is that a woman reports noticing a lack of movement from her baby near to the end of an often uneventful pregnancy.' Zoe goes on to say that the world 'falls apart' when no heartbeat can be found and an ultrasound confirms the baby has died. All of a sudden there are discussions taking place about how the baby will be born – born sleeping.[1]

Michelle Galilee, Sydney-based doula and grief counsellor describes herself as a mother of four in her arms and six in her heart after losing six pregnancies to miscarriage.

'When we lost our first baby, it was probably the first time my husband had witnessed me in such a vulnerable place. Until this point in our relationship I had been a superwoman with big plans and not much could break me. Miscarriage and stillbirth did. And we didn't know it then, but loss was to visit our family five more times,' says Michelle.

After a woman gives birth, her body responds in the same physical ways, whether the baby survives or not. 'The physical reality of pregnancy loss, early term, mid term or late term, is never discussed. Nobody told me that I would produce milk and my breasts would ache to feed a baby,' says Michelle. 'The doctors never mentioned that I would feel after-birth pains and that I would bleed much like I had just given birth. Nobody mentioned that a drop in hormone levels causes a baby blues-like sadness that isn't just over the loss of your baby, but more like a hormonal car crash that everyone stops to watch, but nobody understands.'

For some men, the grief of a lost child is expressed in a very different way from their partner and this can be difficult to navigate as a couple.

'The emotional reality for me was a very dark one. Every single time I lost a baby I wondered why my husband could get up and go to work, but I couldn't summon the courage to go outside. I could feel and appreciate his nurturing of me during this time, but I resented it that he could just go on like nothing had happened. I waited patiently for it to hit him that our baby was gone. That he had to take down the cot and pack up the nursery. But he never did.

'Eight months after we lost our little boy, someone very close to us had a baby,' says Michelle. 'I asked my husband to come with me to a baby store we'd visited during that last pregnancy and his reaction astonished me. He said that he wasn't ready to go back there again and needed some more time to grieve our lost baby. I had almost completely recovered, yet he was still holding on.'

As a doula, Michelle's work has led her to support couples through the birth of a stillborn baby. One of her clients brought her 39 week antenatal appointment forward because she couldn't feel her baby kick anymore and Michelle was there with her when she discovered that her baby had died in utero.

'It was heartbreaking as I held her hand while the midwife moved the doppler over her abdomen, searching for a heart beat,' says Michelle. 'At first there was a reassuring joke about how this happens all the time, bub is probably hiding somewhere. But after a few minutes the energy in the room became one of panic and I struggled to stay strong to support my client. An ultrasound confirmed that the baby had inexplicably died. I frantically tried to get hold of her husband as she sat frozen in a room with a pot plant, two chairs and a box of tissues on a table.'

Michelle goes on to describe what the following days and weeks were like for that couple: 'My client's husband, grief stricken and in shock, did not cry that day. All day he sat and held his partner's hand while she cried, screamed and shook, giving birth to her baby. As their baby came into the world asleep, he stayed strong for her. He stroked her head, rubbed her back, took photos and kept friends and family up to date.

'In the last hours before their baby boy was taken to the morgue, I helped the two of them bathe and dress their little boy. We took more photos and foot and hand prints for them to keep as tangible evidence that their baby had existed. I witnessed two people mourn and cope in such completely different ways, yet they supported each other in every sense.

'At the funeral a week later my client confided to me that although the week had been devastating and a time that as a couple they would never forget, she had experienced a beautiful and intimate week with her partner. They had cried together. They had really talked for the first time in ages. They had become angry together and had gone on long walks on the beach discussing what their future looked like, now that they were to remain two and not three. Losing a baby changes people – it changes relationships too.'

In rare cases, the baby dies during labour or very shortly after with the outcome being a terrible shock. In these cases, couples have no time to prepare for such an outcome and the grief can be overwhelming.

If you and your partner are told that your baby has died in the womb, there will be practical and physical changes to the way that your baby will be born. Take some time, if you have it, to discuss how you would like your baby's entry into the world to be, who will be present, and what memories the two of you would like to make.

Making these memories can be bitter sweet. The birth of a child is such a momentous event that parents want to record every moment. But when that child is stillborn, you may not feel that you will want to remember what may feel like the worst day of your life. Honouring the memory of the birth of your baby who will not go home in your arms seems too much to bear, yet this little one has been such a big part of your life and your dreams for the future. The following page lists some ways to make memories in the short term and things that you might want to do later, after the shock of your loss has subsided.

A friend, family member or a doula can be invaluable during the loss of a baby and in the aftermath. A good support person will ensure that you and your partner are able to focus on each other and on the formalities of the hours and days ahead. Choose someone who can be sensitive to your needs, who can give you both time alone to grieve, and somebody who has experience and wisdom around loss.

Give your partner the physical support that she needs at each stage of the loss. It may be that she requires a heat pack to be warmed regularly, or she may forget to eat or drink due to shock. Although you will have

Memory making
- *Take prints of your baby's hands and feet*
- *Keep a lock of your baby's hair*
- *Publish a birth announcement which includes your baby's name, birth date and that your baby was born peacefully sleeping*
- *Take photos of your baby after the birth, during cuddles and while bathing and dressing. Some photographers and artists specialise in taking photos or painting babies who have died.*
- *Plant a garden or a tree for your baby. If you are renting or if you move often, you could plant a small tree that is potted and can be moved when you vacate.*
- *Give your partner a piece of jewellery which bears your baby's initial. She will then carry with her symbolically the child who is not in her arms.*
- *Keep a memory box with photos, the blanket that your baby was wrapped in and all other mementos. This may be the only proof that your baby did exist and something that you and your partner can keep to signify your short time with him or her. It is also good for future children to have something that they can touch and see and to create a connection with.*

the same emotional feelings, you will not be dealing with the physical ones. This will be one of the most traumatic experiences of her life and she will be faced with the same physical aspects of birth (be it vaginal birth or Caesarean section) and the same physical aspects postnatally. You may need to remember to give her prescribed medications on discharge from hospital. Or you may need to take care of the practical side of life for her indefinitely, arranging time off work for both of you, ensuring shopping and housekeeping is taken care of, seeking childcare for other children if you have them.

Don't forget to take care of yourself. Take time out when you can and think about what this loss means for you and how you are going to get through it. Talk to someone about what is happening to you and your partner. This person may be a friend, a hospital social worker, a kind nurse or midwife, or someone you might never have considered until the moment comes. Remember to take breaks and eat, drink and sleep when you can.

Give your partner space when she wants and needs it, and be there when she needs you. It's a fine balance. Grief has no set pattern and unfortunately there is no manual. You will need to trust your intuition when it comes to this, especially if your partner is feeling extremely vulnerable and is unable to voice her needs and wants.

It may be some time before your partner feels she can face other people or talk about the loss. In the early days after a baby dies, often those around you assume that you have had a live baby. There will be times when you will need to tell those people what has happened. People often do not know how to communicate or respond to new parents when a baby has died. It might be easier for you to tell those close to you about your loss right away and deal with people of lesser significance later on. Sometimes an email to those people with basic details and information on when you and your partner will be in contact again can help those around you to communicate better with you and your partner. Perhaps asking a family member or trusted friend to pass on that information on your behalf might be helpful until you and your partner are able to discuss your loss with others.

After the loss of a baby, it may seem natural or instinctive to mention 'trying again'. Your partner may talk about this straight away. Or she may not mention it for several weeks, months or years. You will also have your own feelings about this and you may not know how you feel about it for some time. Talk to each other about another baby when the time is right for you both.

Nothing can really prepare you for the loss of a baby but these pointers may help in some way:

- *Support your partner in all the usual physical ways to give birth*
- *Spend some time with your baby, take photos and cuddle*
- *Pull in a good support person to help you and your partner*
- *Look after yourself too and find someone to talk this through with*
- *Recognise from the outset that you and your partner may grieve very differently and that's OK*
- *Talk about the possibility of trying again when the time is right*

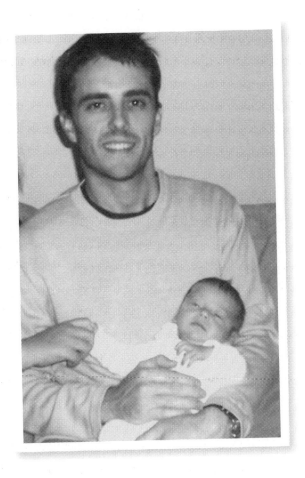

DAVID GALILEE'S STORY

Thankfully, our surviving babies were stubborn fighters who fought for every breath and slowly grew into strong and healthy children.

David Galilee was studying for a science degree in zoology when he met his wife Michelle at the annual Sydney University Science Ball. He became an aquarist at Sydney Aquarium before moving on to become a zookeeper at Taronga Zoo. Caring for animals required hours that weren't ideal for family life, so David changed career direction and moved to the Australian Quarantine and Inspection Service as a quarantine inspector. David is father to four school-aged children (Katie, Sophie, Aimee and Jack) and foster dad to many as emergency and short-term foster care placements. However, this Sydney couple has suffered six miscarriages – losses that have had far-reaching effects on them both. But life goes on and Dave recently drove a motorhome from Sydney to Alice Springs and back with Michelle and all four kids. He looks forward to a future full of motorhome adventures, quality time with his family and caring for more foster kids. David has not, does not, and never will understand the mind of a teenage girl.

My wife and I have four children. The older two babies were blessed with natural births and Michelle experienced no complications. The younger two were less fortunate. Their pregnancies were cursed with serious complications, countless threatened miscarriages and traumatic premature births by emergency high-risk Caesareans.

Our daughter Aimee was born at 27 weeks due to undiagnosed placental abruptions [*where the placenta separates from the uterus*]. I remember following my wife's ambulance in our car as she was transferred from our local hospital to one with a specialist nursery then leaving her that night to go home to our other two children. When I went back to the hospital the next morning Michelle had spent the night in another ward due to seizures and an irregular heart beat. That afternoon, our third child Aimee was born.

It was a blur of consent forms and surgeons. As my wife was wheeled away to theatre, I was given a hurried and frantic tour of the nursery, where I waited alone in the tiny parents' room. Time seemed to stand still and then suddenly the room came alive with activity. My tiny daughter was wheeled in and the staff began working on her. From behind the small group of doctors and midwives, I watched the controlled chaos as a midwife attempted to explain what was happening. To this day I have no idea what she said to me.

The trauma of the event was very difficult to cope with. For my wife, however, it was sheer hell. While recovering from the physical and emotional trauma of an emergency Caesarean, she somehow needed to find the strength for daily visits to the hospital and to be a mother to our other two young children.

When a baby is born this early, nobody quite knows how to react. Friends and family are subdued and cautious. The concept of 'congratulations' which usually accompanies a birth is conspicuously absent. Nobody wants to commit to a celebration without first knowing that the outcome will be positive.

For me, I consciously attempted to fill this void. I never allowed myself to consider that our daughter would not survive. Even as other babies in the nursery quietly died, I would not let my wife lose hope. Physically and mentally, hope was all that kept us going. Our daughter remained in hospital for nearly four months and eventually, we took her home and she grew healthy and strong!

Four years later, Michelle had another tough pregnancy. Complications were evident very early on. She was told she had miscarried, but was convinced that she was still pregnant. Obstetricians, ultrasound technicians and GPs were all convinced that we had lost the baby. Through all this, Michelle was resolute that there was still a baby inside wanting to be heard. Before the scheduled curettage, she demanded a final ultrasound, which discovered a tiny heartbeat.

She had miscarried one twin, but had still sensed another clinging to life inside. Had we listened to the experts, we would not have our son Jack today. From this experience, I learnt to have more faith in my wife's intuition and began to question the absolute trust that I had placed in the medical fraternity.

Michelle was diagnosed with placenta praevia [*where the placenta grows over the cervix*] and was told to rest as much as possible. There were threatened miscarriages and the fear of haemorrhage, which could have rapidly claimed the life of my wife and our baby. In the end she was sent to hospital for total bed rest.

The stress was unbelievable but there were still small celebrations. Every day that we managed to keep our baby in the womb felt like a major milestone. After our experiences with a premature baby, we were prepared for an early delivery and celebrated quietly as we managed 24 weeks gestation and then 27. We were now in familiar territory and knew that if our son was born he could have a good chance of survival.

My role at this time was to help combat the extreme boredom my wife felt while on total bed rest for six weeks. If I arrived to visit without a bundle of the latest trashy magazines, I knew I was in trouble. I was also the sole provider of edible food. Six weeks of hospital food definitely took a toll on my wife's mental health.

Finally, a date was set for a Caesarean. The doctor talked to us both and discussed the risks. Again, I was determined to remain positive. The magnitude of having to say our goodbyes and get her affairs in order prior to surgery has still never really hit home. It was at this time that I needed to be at my strongest.

Thankfully, despite needing a blood transfusion, the surgery went well, our baby boy was born and once again the cycle of new parenthood continued.

At times Michelle found it hard to cope after such a difficult pregnancy and traumatic birth. She was often angry with me because she thought I was lucky to go to work. I hated leaving my family and certainly did not feel lucky. It was extremely difficult to get on stage and present the Seal Show with a carefree smile on my face, when internally I was a bundle of stress and nerves, feeling terribly guilty for having to leave my wife and children at home.

Somehow, we managed to get through it and the experience has ultimately brought us closer as a couple and as a family. In time, I also found a new job with a healthier approach to balancing family and career.

Overall we have been very lucky to have four beautiful children, but we have not always been so fortunate. Along the way, we have lost six babies.

As a father, my experiences with pregnancy loss have varied in emotion and trauma as they have occurred during different periods of my life. As a young man in my early and mid-twenties, the miscarriages involved feelings of loss and grief, but I considered my role to be there to provide physical and emotional support for my wife. We were young and healthy so there was always more time to try again. I was busy building a career and had distractions to keep me from dwelling on our loss. In my quiet times (which were few) I would occasionally think about what might have been, but most of the time I pushed those feelings to the back of my mind and just got on with it.

After several early miscarriages in rapid succession, our doctor decided that we should undergo some genetic testing. There were lots of probing questions and blood tests. One bleak overcast day as we waited for results, the tension in the room was excruciating. I saw an old defibrillator in the corner, quickly grabbed the panels, put them on my head, and yelled, 'Clear!' In hindsight, this was probably a pretty dangerous attempt at humour, but Michelle laughed and the mood in the room shifted from tense and foreboding, to relaxed and almost lighthearted.

I've always used humour to break tension and act as a distraction to a stressful or scary situation. Sometimes my jokes have the opposite effect and are misinterpreted as insensitive, but overall I'd say humour has helped us as a couple to get through some pretty dark times. Neonatal intensive care wards can be depressing. Without a sense of humour, I don't think we could have coped at all.

Our last miscarriage was by far the most difficult for me. I'd had a vasectomy several years earlier so this pregnancy was entirely unexpected. My feelings were mixed. As the pregnancy progressed incident free, and my wife's good health continued, my feelings gradually shifted from sheer terror, to begrudging acceptance, to cautious optimism.

I felt myself slowly beginning to look forward to another baby. Plans changed, names were considered, and we began to shop for baby things. It wasn't long before I was fully absorbed in the idea of another baby. The miscarriage came suddenly and knocked both of us off our feet. I went to work one day thinking of my impending fatherhood, received a frantic text message and left work to meet my wife at our GP's rooms. By then it was all over and all the plans I was beginning to make, and look forward to, had disappeared.

My wife was devastated and I did my best to support her. Despite my previous experiences of coping with a miscarriage, I was overwhelmed with emotions and caught severely off guard by the magnitude of grief and loss. I tried to be strong and dealt with most of my feelings internally. Those feelings are still there, almost as strong. Even after many months,

I find it difficult to think about and even now, I can't walk into a baby store as it stirs up too many emotions and feelings that I haven't been able to deal with yet.

Despite all the support I have tried to provide for Michelle and all the experiences we have shared, I still have no genuine understanding of how she has felt during and after each pregnancy. As men, we just don't have the capacity to fully empathise with our partners. We can try to imagine how it must feel to fall pregnant, give birth, or suffer a miscarriage, but ultimately we can only draw upon our own individual experiences and our imagination to try and piece together what it must be like for them.

The difficulty has always been that men do not have any physical attachment to a pregnancy. We don't experience any of the physical or hormonal changes that a pregnancy brings to our partner or the physical changes that come with miscarriage. Most miscarriages occur behind closed doors and men are rarely involved. Maybe this is a bad thing. We have a huge investment of emotions and feelings for something that we have never seen or felt. This makes it very difficult to grieve and feel closure.

These days, parents of late term stillborn babies are encouraged to hold the baby, take photos and say goodbye. This may help with the grieving process. For the parents of babies who miscarry early in the pregnancy, this is not possible. The mother feels the physical and emotional pain associated with the loss, but the father is more removed. We don't really know how to feel. This can be a good thing as it means we can focus on helping our partners, but often results in the incorrect perception that we don't care or are not suffering in our own way. This is particularly true if you are prone to using off-beat humour, like me.

Thankfully, our two youngest children were stubborn fighters who fought for every breath and grew into strong and healthy children. Today, they can still be incredibly stubborn and a major pain in the arse! Sometimes, when they are at their least likeable, I have to remind myself that possessing these character traits may very well have given them the strength to survive.

CHAPTER 7

HOW TO BE AN ADVOCATE FOR YOUR FAMILY

Now is the time for you to start fending for your child and protecting your family as a father. This role really begins when your partner becomes pregnant and you start avoiding childbirth horror stories and the judgements that other people may place on your childbirth choices.

When it comes to the birth, however, you will need to step up as your partner's advocate. She won't be in a position to bat for herself, no matter how confident and feisty she might usually be. I'm the vocal one in our relationship but I really needed Bruce to take over when I was in labour. On the day your partner gives birth, she will use all her energy to birth her baby, so she needs you to be the spokesperson for the family when she is in the world of birth.

Fourteen reconstructive operations to put me back together after a motorcycle accident taught me a valuable lesson about hospitals. Most medical caregivers go about their job with professionalism and care but you have to live with the fall-out if there is a catastrophic failure. You have the most to lose so you'd better step up and look out for yourself and your loved ones.

In my case, I am the only one who has had to live with spectacular scars and physical limitations after the failure of several experimental procedures at the hands of a team of gung-ho surgeons. I completely surrendered myself to their expert, senior care. In retrospect, this was a mistake.

By about my tenth operation I had clued-in to the fact that these surgeons were experimenting. On my limbs! I had allowed them to try ludicrous operations that had me in theatre for ten hours at a time, taking veins and muscles and skin from all over my body and grafting them to one traumatised site. In the end, the procedure that worked (and saved the leg I was about to lose) was a procedure that doctors have been using since World War II. No one offered me the tried and true method at the start. I should have *asked*. If I'd fully understood the options available and the risks involved, I'd have avoided four or five complicated operations and some pretty hideous scars.

Once I switched gear and realised that I was the only one who was going to fend for me and the limb I was going to have to live with for the rest of my life, I was my own advocate. I started reading my own medical notes, asking lots of questions, borrowing text books from surgeons and being a regular pest.

When you are in hospital, your medical notes are about you, so you have every right to read them. I had time to kill so I asked the nurses to teach me how to read the charts and their nursing shorthand. Once I had some knowledge, I could ask the right questions and make better decisions on my care. These weren't medical emergencies, they were choices or preferences about my care. I am a very different patient now from the one I was in those first months in hospital.

You may not think of your partner as a patient when she gives birth but if you have chosen to birth in a hospital, that's exactly what she is. She is part of a hospital system that is responsible for her health, but she is the one who has to live with the consequences if the system fails.

Don't be afraid to ask what might be perceived as dumb questions and to ask for clarification if you don't understand the answers. Enquire and pursue until you are satisfied that you understand what's going on and how your caregivers are managing the health of your partner.

I supported a couple once and the expectant dad was a plumber. He was worried about all the 'choices' that had been mentioned in the hospital antenatal classes. 'I'm a plumber,' he said to me, 'but I know very little about female plumbing and I'm worried about making all these decisions during the labour that are out of my league.'

If it's a medical emergency, you'll know about it but you won't be making those sorts of choices. In fact, if there is a medical emergency and you hamper the care of your partner and child, for example, by refusing an emergency Caesarean, you'll be required to sign medical indemnity forms to absolve the hospital of responsibility.

Hospitals are big businesses that have to run to set protocols for safety, efficiency and profitability. However, some hospital protocols are flexible so you should know the difference between what is standard hospital procedure and what is a medical necessity. Some things are procedural and can be negotiated if you ask, while others are about the health of the baby and are not negotiable.

For example, most public hospitals will allow your partner to go seven to ten days over your estimated due date. However, if you ask for daily monitoring and regular ultrasounds, your caregivers may be willing to let you go to 14 days or more over your estimated due date in order to avoid an induction. You won't know unless you ask.

Some protocols are defined by your partner's obstetrician, if you have engaged one, while others are defined by the hospital. For example, the obstetrician will decide if you can have an extra person, such as your doula, in theatre for a Caesarean, but it is usually hospital protocol that dictates how long a patient must remain in recovery before she is returned to the ward. You won't know unless you investigate, so ask questions and negotiate from there. You may want to go to recovery with your partner and baby after a Caesarean. This isn't the usual protocol but there's nothing to stop you from asking.

Hospitals can be intimidating to those without a medical background. Remember that you are the customer in this situation so don't feel intimidated by hospital personnel. This is their workplace and they are confident here, but this is your birth suite to use and you have paid for it. I don't mean that you should treat the midwife like a waiter but don't let staff treat you like a trespasser either.

As soon as you are given your birth suite, familiarise yourself with it. See Chapter 9 for a full list of what to do when you arrive at the hospital to make yourself at home and your partner at ease. Make the space yours and know your way around it.

When dealing with your caregivers, ask what the downsides are for whatever intervention is being offered. For example, your partner's caregiver may say, 'Let's pop her on a drip to kick along labour and have this baby sooner rather than later.' They may put a positive spin on it but they probably won't mention that a Syntocinon drip produces unnaturally painful contractions and that most women beg for an epidural soon after they begin. Ask about the pros and cons and request time alone as a couple to decide. Don't feel pushed to make quick decisions about your preferences.

Most midwives are wonderful, compassionate, professional people who want to work with women and babies. I have met only one or two who should be working in the morgue rather than with live patients. However, while this might be the biggest day in your life, it's just another shift for the midwife. Don't expect them to shower you with petals. They have a job to do and a baby to deliver in the next room too.

Use the midwives' names, be polite and considerate and they will do their best to look after you and your partner well. Being demanding or aggressive won't make you popular with your caregivers and won't help your partner either.

Handle any conflict with your caregivers with adrenalin in mind. If you're having a bingle with the midwife, you could make your partner anxious and this will produce adrenalin, which will slow down the birth process and make it more painful. If you absolutely have to, take the discussion outside the room, but remember that this will leave your partner alone.

'I know of a case where the father was so agitated and felt so threatened that he punched the midwife,' says Hannah Dahlen, Associate Professor of Midwifery at the University of Western Sydney and a midwife with over twenty years of baby-catching experience prior to her academic career. 'It's the ugly side of a primitive streak we see where men respond to the adrenalin and testosterone that's wildly flowing in their body and the loss of control or threat to their wife and baby can make them erupt.'

Hannah says she has witnessed men barricade the room with furniture, barring all caregivers from entering.

These are extreme cases and Hannah says that it takes a skilful midwife to be able to identify early on that there may be an 'eruption' and to act quickly to make this man feel supported and not threatened.

Non-English speaking men may feel even more threatened, says Hannah, because they can't always understand what is going on. Bilingual health workers can support these couples and telephone interpreters are available.

'Unfortunately, some midwives love a fight,' says Hannah. 'They see the birth unit as their territory and anyone threatening their turf should be dealt with. The least amount of conflict appears to be where the woman, her partner and the midwife have a chance to get to know each other before the birth and develop a trusting relationship. You hardly ever see conflict in these models of care because there is lots of open communication and trust. Without trust nothing works in birth.'

Communication is the key; talk to the midwife courteously and clearly. Ask for more information and don't feel pushed by a stroppy caregiver.

If you feel threatened or unheard, make these feelings clear. Make it easy for your partner's caregivers to meet your needs by communicating what those needs are. Midwives are not mind readers. For example, 'I feel like this situation is getting out of control and I need you to slow down and explain to me what is happening here.'

If you are verbally or physically abusive or threatening in any way to staff or your partner, you'll be escorted off the premises by a security guard who's a lot bigger and tougher than you are. So keep your cool. Remember that making your partner stressed will make her labour harder and if you're twiddling your thumbs in the car park after being booted out, you're hardly helping her give birth. And an assault charge wouldn't be a good start to fatherhood.

If you have a midwife you believe is hampering the progress of the birth, you need to see the Nursing Unit Manager and ask for a different midwife to be assigned to you and your partner.

I have never personally seen conflict between a couple and their caregivers escalate to this point, but it happens from time to time, so be aware that you can ask for a different caregiver or you can just wait out the shift for a new midwife to come on duty.

Remember that you are the spokesperson for your family, not the Minister of Defence. You don't have to go into combat mode to be able to protect your partner and baby effectively.

To be the best advocate for your partner, remember the following points:

- *You are the defender of the birthplace and the spokesperson for your family*
- *While medical personnel may do their best, it is you, your partner and your baby who will have to live with the consequences if there is a catastrophic failure, so ask questions and understand the medical side of what's on offer*
- *Know the difference between hospital protocol and medical necessity*
- *Make yourself at home in the birth suite and don't feel intimidated*
- *Take your time to make decisions alone as a couple*
- *Handle conflict with your partner's adrenalin in mind*

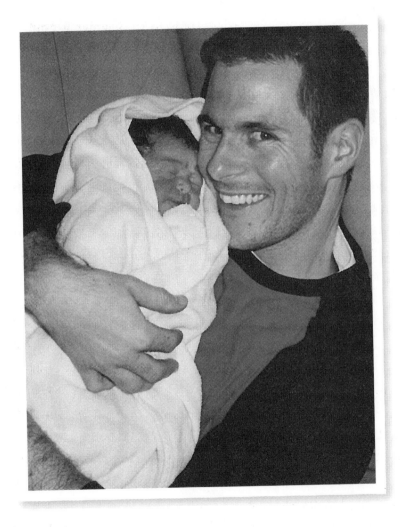

DIGBY HONE'S STORY

I continue to believe that guys were not built to have babies and put up with that level of pain.

Dr Digby Hone fell in love with and married a widow with three young children when he was in his final year of a medicine degree at Sydney University. He and Liza went on to have two children of their own. Digby is now a qualified paediatric emergency specialist working in the casualty department of three major hospitals and is the only emergency specialist to pass his final exams as the father of five children. His training saw him working in anaesthetics, administering epidurals on the labour ward and spinal blocks for Caesareans in theatre, places where he saw many fathers face their role in childbirth, some not as well as others. Then it was his turn...

My wife's first husband died of cancer within about three months of his initial diagnosis. Liza was left with three little kids aged one, five and seven. We met a few months after Greg died and we got together about a year after that, after much heartache on my part, trying to work out how I would be a boyfriend, and eventually a husband, to a woman with three little kids.

Adapting to being an instant father was a huge challenge. Sometimes when things were difficult, I would wonder what Greg would do in that situation, but they're great kids and despite our troubles, they've embraced me as their dad and I really love them. I never refer to them as my step-kids, they're just my kids, all of them. Becky is the eldest, then Alex and Gus. Liza and I then had two children together, Jasmine and Cooper. I hoped that having kids of my own would teach me even more about how to connect more closely with and love all my kids.

Before I asked Liza to marry me I wanted to know whether she would be prepared to have more children and whether that would even be anatomically possible! She was willing and able. We knew we wouldn't be losing lifestyle or opportunities if we had more kids. We were already in the thick of it. We had just settled into our new house when Liza got pregnant with Jasmine. It was fantastic.

I felt at ease knowing that Liza was a very experienced mother and had given birth three times already. Liza's first three babies had been born close to their due dates and she'd had very rapid labours. She'd have little or no warning, with contractions starting very close together and then she would give birth soon after. Though quick, her first and second labours were incredibly painful and I couldn't believe that she was willing to go through all that again for me. Some women love being pregnant but Liza hated it and found it harder and harder each time.

About a month before Jasmine was due I had made plans to go up to our farm with some mates. A friend has his commercial pilot's licence and so we were flying there, about a two-hour flight to the New England area. When we were taking off there was a lot of cloud. I remember praying, 'God, if Jazzy is not supposed to come now, please part the clouds so we can go.' We had an awesome weekend. Coming home, there was storm activity again, but we made it home by 8pm and Liza started contractions about half an hour later.

Her contractions started as Braxton Hicks, more like tightenings. The World Cup Cricket Final between Australia and Pakistan was on and I thought the tightenings were just because Liza was excited about the cricket but she thought it was because she was happy that I'd made it home safely from the farm.

We watched the cricket until about midnight, while these tightenings continued, but they weren't painful at all. Liza didn't think she was in labour yet, so I examined her and found she was four centimetres dilated. I had done a ten-week obstetrics and gynaecology term while Liza was pregnant so I had had a bit of experience in this.

Liza called the hospital and the midwife had a good go at Liza, saying, 'This is your fourth child, you should know if you're in labour or not!' with Liza saying to her, 'Well no, it doesn't feel like the others.' We were amazed that it seemed a different father brought different labour experiences.

We watched another hour of cricket and then we thought it would be a good idea to help bring on labour more strongly so we had sex and we think this broke her waters. The contractions became more regular so we went into the hospital.

Unfortunately we got the midwife we'd spoken to on the phone. She was a nightmare. She was very blunt and we felt quite unsupported. I think she didn't like it that I was a doctor. When we arrived I said, 'My wife's five centimetres dilated,' and the midwife didn't like that much. I asked Liza to see if we could turn on the TV for the end of the cricket. Fortunately the midwife allowed us to, despite being cranky about it.

When Liza was seven centimetres dilated she still had almost nonexistent contraction pain. We were making jokes and were thrilled when Australia won the World Cup final. With the cricket over, Liza decided it was time to get on with it and we knew the second stage of labour was going to be frighteningly fast.

Our obstetrician, Dr Rod Kirsop, was called in and arrived looking half asleep. Admittedly, it was 2am and I felt bad for getting him out of bed at that hour. Rod is an ex-professional surfer and had surfed with the likes of Mark Occhilupo on the Pro Tour in the '80s. The year before he delivered my daughter, he'd won a big wave surfing title in Hawaii.

Rod and the midwife were talking about the new surgical gloves with their backs turned to us. Rod had one glove on and the other only half on, when I looked down and saw Jazzy's head starting to appear. I said, 'Rod, quick!' and with the next contraction Jasmine's head popped out.

The second stage of labour had been only about seven minutes long and was relatively painless until those last few minutes.

I had been concerned that I wouldn't be able to connect emotionally with our baby when she was born. I'm a person who is led by the heart but when it comes to medical stuff I often keep a level of emotional disconnection. Despite this, I burst into tears when I held Jasmine for the first time. Whenever I told anyone about her birth, I would tear up. I remember driving home crying. It was a huge release, with a flood of tears and emotion.

Cooper's birth was quite different from Jasmine's. We thought he'd be even quicker but his birth was quite prolonged and a lot more painful for Liza.

One night, at about the 37-week mark, I got home from Emergency at about 1am and found Liza still up. She said, 'We're having this baby tonight!' She didn't have any contractions at that point, just determination to have this baby. We had some hot sex as another attempt to manipulate the situation and get labour started. Sure enough…

Once we got to hospital, we couldn't believe it – we had the same midwife! She tried to send us home, telling Liza she wasn't yet in established labour, but we stayed. There were a couple of hours when Liza had a sleep and I had a snooze on the couch. At some stage I jokingly offered to put in an epidural and the midwife nearly bit my head off. 'No you won't!' she said. Liza got the joke.

Cooper's birth was much more painful and it was difficult to see Liza in such pain. I kept turning up the gas and did all I could to help her. It was beneficial for me to have seen a number of guys being supportive to their wives in the past. I stayed close, held her hand, rubbed her back and communicated with her so I could see how she was feeling.

As part of my training I did a year of anaesthetics as well as an obstetrics and gynaecology term so I have seen over a hundred Caesareans. It's pretty weird when you've given a woman a spinal for a Caesarean and she's having her abdomen cut open, just chatting away without feeling any pain from what's going on below.

There were times when I was called to give an epidural to a woman in labour but found that she was too advanced to have one safely. It's incredibly difficult to keep the patient still when contractions are so close together. Some women hold out for the doctor to get there to put in their epidural and when you have to say no, you'll get death stares, but then ten or twenty minutes later they've delivered their baby.

Sometimes a midwife will call me and say, 'This woman is asking for an epidural but she's progressing nicely so can you just take your time?'

Some fathers just don't know what to do with themselves at the birth. They sit well away from their partner with no affection or touching. Their wife is in pain and they have no idea how to help. Theatre is definitely a daunting place. As the anaesthetist, I would encourage them along a bit and say, 'Come on, come and sit right here and hold her hand,' and sit them right next to their wife.

I've had two guys who passed out in theatre. I'd told them the baby was about to be delivered and they'd got up to have a quick look and over they went! Initially we have other more urgent issues to deal with so we just have to leave them on the floor.

The very first baby I delivered as a med student was with a young couple. The girl was only about 19 and she had been in labour for about 20 hours. I walked in and there was this girl walking around the room stark naked and howling with each contraction. Her parents were there, her dad had a video camera, as did her husband. She would contract while squatting and they'd put a mirror under her to show her how well she was doing. They were videoing right into the mirror saying, 'We'll have to show this at the baby's 21st!' I couldn't believe the circus in there.

I continue to believe that guys were not built to have babies and put up with that level of pain. I see that every day with men in pain in the emergency department. You get some stoic men but on the whole you see a lot more bravery from women in putting up with pain. Men tend to deal poorly with pain.

After being with her for both Jasmine and Cooper's births, I look at Liza with a new sense of respect, admiration and love.

Being a father has helped me to relate better to the parents who bring their children into Emergency. I think it gives me a bit more credibility with these people when I tell them I'm a father of five. I used to find babies crying at work really annoying before I had my own babies. Not any more.

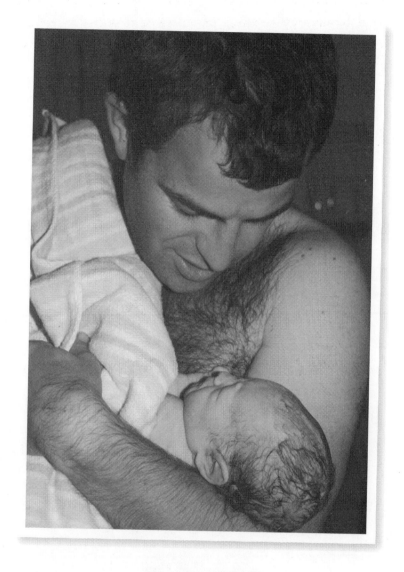

PART TWO

CHAPTER 8
PRELABOUR

The next five chapters will take you through each stage of a typical first labour, giving you specific practical tips on what to do and when, in order to support your partner well and engage in the birth in a positive, hands-on way. These chapters will also prepare you for what to expect from a woman and her typical behaviour in labour. There is also a chapter on what to expect and what is expected of you, if your partner has a Caesarean. Thirty percent of you will face that challenge.

There are two terms you need to understand, otherwise the next few chapters won't make much sense: contractions and cervical dilation.

The uterus is a giant muscle that expands to 600 times its usual size when your partner is full term. Contractions in labour are tightenings of this muscle, tightenings that effectively bring the baby down and push the baby out. The uterus only gets a few gigs its whole life and performs amazingly well for a muscle that can't go to the gym.

The cervix lies between the top of the vagina and the base of the uterus. This amazing little piece of anatomy has to dilate or open up to let your baby through the birth canal. Dilation is measured in centimetres and the magic number is ten. You want your partner to be ten centimetres dilated before she can start pushing your baby out.

Prelabour is the warm-up phase of labour when your partner will start to feel contractions. These are not just tightenings, or Braxton Hicks contractions as they are called, but contracting of the uterus that registers some pain. The cervix softens and shortens with some degree of dilation.

Prelabour is gentle and your partner will be able to speak during contractions and will probably still be calling the shots. It can last just a couple of hours or it can go on for days so stay close by and preferably don't go to work. Start making final preparations for this birth.

Penny Simkins, author of *The Birth Partner*, an American book that has become the global doula bible, refers to a childbirth support person as the 'guardian of the birth place'[1]. You need to start the role of guardian and protector as soon as your partner is in prelabour.

Ideally, you'll have a flexible arrangement with your employer that allows you to take paternity or annual leave starting on the day that your partner goes into labour. This means you don't have to guess when your baby will arrive when applying for leave (only 3% of babies arrive on their estimated due date) and you won't waste precious annual leave entitlements playing the waiting game. It's common for first babies to go a little overdue, but don't bank on that. Your partner will need you much more after your baby is born, than before the birth.

Some women don't experience a prelabour stage at all and dive straight into the main event with painful contractions close together. If this is the case, you won't have time to pack. You won't have time to do much else at all, as you'll be needed to help your partner manage each contraction (review Chapter 5 for pain management strategies).

If you haven't already packed for hospital, do so now. My friend Leon told me about the birth of his first child, which was extremely sudden. 'All I can say is, make sure you've packed for hospital by the 36 week mark!' said Leon. He and his wife were taken by surprise when their baby came early with an emergency Caesarean, which didn't give Leon any time to prepare for hospital.

Some women feel less anxious when they know they are packed and ready and they can just walk out the door when they need to. If putting the bags in the car will make her feel more at ease, then do that.

Packing list for you

- Snacks – such as cheese sandwiches, bag of snakes, fruit and nut mix, muesli bars, energy bars
- Water – sports drinks have extra salts and sugars in them
- Breath mints and deodorant – remember, you will be unpopular if you stink
- Swimmers – to get into the bath or shower with your partner
- Socks – hospitals get cold
- Thongs – you're not allowed to wander around the hospital with bare feet and you may be in and out of the shower or bath
- MP3 player with a ten-hour birth playlist and speakers
- Your pain management tool kit: essential oils, labour massage oil, heat packs, visual focus
- Camera and video camera with fully charged batteries
- A copy of your birth plan if you have written one
- A change of clothes

What NOT to pack

- Your laptop or anything to do with work
- The novel you are reading or the newspaper
- Any other kind of entertainment device (other than for birth music)
- Your mother

Packing list for your partner

- Lip balm or Vaseline
- Comfortable pyjamas for her to wear once the baby is born
- Things to make the birth suite feel more like home, such as her pillow
- One pack of Depend incontinence underwear – great for the first few days of postnatal bleeding and no washing for you to take home
- Toiletries bag: toothbrush and toothpaste, hairbrush, moisturiser
- Socks, maternity bra and clothes to go home in

Packing list for your baby

- Jump suits x 3, appropriate for the time of year
- Baby bonnet if the weather is cold
- Newborn nappies x 1 pack
- Baby wipes
- Baby wraps x 3

You must have a car seat fitted properly in your car before you can take your baby home so it's best to have this done before your partner goes into labour. My brother rocked up to take his wife and baby home with the baby seat still in its cardboard box. His wife stood in the car park holding the baby while he battled to install it and in the end my sister-in-law said, 'Here, take the baby and I'll do it!' It's best to have this sorted out well before the birth. Some hospitals offer a child restraint fitting service.

Once you are packed for hospital, call your caregivers and let them know what's happening. If your partner's waters have broken, your caregivers will want to know what colour the fluid is. If it is clear or pink, they will probably want you to stay at home until contractions are closer together. If the fluid is green or black, this indicates that your baby has passed meconium, its first poo. This can be an indication of distress in your baby so your caregivers may want you to come in to the hospital straight away to monitor the baby.

Remember that most public hospitals in Australia will give you about 24 hours from the time waters break to the time they want you to start labour. This is to prevent infection, because the amniotic sac has been broken and may let in bacteria. You can usually bargain with your caregivers for more time as long as there is no medical reason to intervene and induce labour.

I don't think it's a good idea to tell people that your partner is in prelabour. Facebook status update? Bad idea. This only puts pressure on your partner to produce your baby within other people's expectations of time. It will also mean that the in-laws might come running and they won't make your job as the primary support person any easier. If you keep this news to yourselves, you'll have the most delicious announcement to make when your baby is born, you won't be pestered with phone calls and text messages from well-meaning family and friends, and you can bunker down and birth this baby in the time it takes.

Talk to your partner about this in the last few weeks before your baby is born and put boundaries in place with family if you have to. Tell them you'll put them in the picture once the baby is born and then you'll have nipped any expectations in the bud. Remember, *this* is your family now and you are their protector.

One of the most common questions I am asked is about when the waters can be expected to break. There's no straight answer for this. A woman's waters can break before she goes into labour, during labour, they can be broken for her by medical intervention and babies can even be born in an intact amniotic sack.

A friend told me about a woman who was approaching her due date and was out to lunch at a swanky outdoor café. Her lunch arrived and she suddenly vomited into her Fettucine Boscaiola! At the same moment, her waters broke and about a litre of amniotic fluid hit the pavement! Poor woman. She said she'll never go back to that café as long as she lives.

When there is a huge downpour of rain and the barometric pressure drops, this can cause waters that are ready to break to go pop.

Sometimes waters breaking can be a trickle and sometimes it seems like a bucketful. As you approach the estimated due date it's recommended that your partner should sit on a couple of towels when she's in the car and that you put a mattress protector on your bed with a few towels underneath it on your partner's side of the bed. A nice new mattress and a few litres of amniotic fluid make for a bit of a disaster.

My friend Barry says that when his wife's waters broke, it felt like an anticlimax and that the upholstery was an asset worth protecting. In his words: 'At about 5am, Andrea's waters broke. That phrase had always brought to mind news footage of levee banks breaking, cattle floating helplessly down the main street and entire towns being inundated. That was the first myth to be busted. It was more like a trickle – so minor a "break" that I accused her of simple incontinence. She apologised. Apparently we were wrong – she had slow-release levee banks. I'm not really an early morning person. Andrea wanted to call the hospital to report the beginning of the deluge but the bed was warm and I was sleepy. With her welfare uppermost in my mind, I said no, don't panic you silly bed-wetter. By 8am, the widening damp patch woke me up and we both went downstairs for breakfast. Now, anyone even vaguely familiar with a 1979 VW Golf will know how pale the seat fabric is. Sure, we were in a rush, but there's always time to protect your assets. So with seven towels on the passenger seat, a bucket in front and her head now scraping the roof lining, we raced to the hospital.'

Back to prelabour. If you have engaged a doula, give her a call to let her know there's some action. You many not need her for hours, or even days, but it will give her a chance to get her life in order so she can be with you when you need her. If your partner starts prelabour in the middle of the night, don't call your doula then. Call her in the morning. She'll be much more useful to you if she's had a good night's sleep. However, if you go into active labour in the middle of the night and you need your doula then, don't hesitate to call her. Calls at 4am are part of the doula gig.

Once I had a call from a doula client at about 2am. The phone is on Bruce's side of the bed and he answered on autopilot as if he were in the office taking a business call, then said, 'Certainly, may I say who's calling?' Who did he think it was at 2am? The bank?

Once you are packed and your caregivers informed, you can focus on your partner. Prelabour can be mind-numblingly boring because there is very little action and it can go on for days.

Encourage your partner to take it easy and rest. It's a bit of a thrill to think that your baby will be born soon, but she needs to resist the urge to use up her energy at this stage of labour. Give her a nice long shoulder massage.

She may not be excited at all. She may be afraid that this is it and she's not ready for it. You have to use calm reassurance and all your manly charm to convince her that she was built to birth, that you'll be with her every step of the way and that you completely adore her. People can achieve great things when they feel loved.

This would be a good time to light a candle in an oil burner or flick the switch on a vaporiser and burn some essential oils to help calm your partner. Childbirth educator, doula and aromatherapist Vickie Hingston-Jones recommends lavender oil for creating a peaceful environment. It is calming and is used as a reliever of pain, a muscle relaxant and anti-depressant. Lavender oil is available from health food stores, vitamin retailers or at your local chemist.

Remember that it is important to use only natural essential oils made from plants and flowers. Synthetic oils, often labelled as fragrant oils, do not contain any therapeutic qualities.

Add four to six drops of lavender oil (lavandula angustifolia) to a vapouriser. Alternatively, add five drops of lavender to 10ml of almond oil and give your partner a relaxing massage to the temples, forehead, upper and lower back and sacrum.

Your partner may enjoy doing distracting things like flipping through photo albums or having you read aloud to her and your baby. Your baby will be familiar with your voice by then.

You could watch a movie but make sure it's something that your partner wants to watch and keep the negative impact of adrenalin in mind. This isn't the time to squeeze in one more rerun of Apocalypse

Now and perhaps you shouldn't flip on the health channel for a few more birth videos. Try a comedy. The movie *Parenthood* might be a good introduction to what the years ahead have in store for you.

Some women become discouraged if prelabour goes on and on. Some books even refer to prelabour as 'false labour', which is hardly useful. Reassure your partner that this is normal progress and that her body is giving her a gentle, natural start. This is a great time for a kiss and a cuddle or even to have sex.

Keep yourself and your partner well fed and hydrated throughout prelabour. Once labour really kicks in, you'll have less time to eat and drink so look after yourselves during this earliest stage.

Monitor contractions to see if you can spot a pattern. A common prelabour pattern could be a contraction every 30 minutes for a few hours and then nothing for an hour, then 15 minutes apart for an hour and then another break.

You should be timing from the beginning of one contraction to the beginning of the next, also noting the length of time for the actual contraction. Your caregivers will probably ask how far apart the contractions are and how long they are lasting.

My friend Justine said her husband thought he was Laurie Lawrence when she was in labour. Mr Clipboard and Stopwatch. He obsessed with timing each contraction, noting a pain ranking out of 10 for each one and then arguing with her about whether it was a 7 or an 8 out of 10! 'You don't want to peak too early!' he said.

Don't get too obsessed with timing contractions – it's not the Olympics. You just need enough information to spot a pattern and see how your partner is progressing.

You are aiming for contractions that are about three or four minutes apart from the start of one to the start of the next, with each contraction lasting a full minute. This is typically when your partner is in active labour, her cervix has started to dilate and the uterus is working hard to contract and bring the baby down. At this point, your partner is in what's referred to as stage one or active labour. This is it!

If your partner has just nudged you awake to tell you she's having contractions every fifteen minutes and you only skim-read this chapter three months ago, these are the important points to remember:

- *Don't go to work*
- *Pack for hospital if you haven't already*
- *Let your caregivers know what's going on*
- *Don't tell people she's in labour*
- *Do distracting things to pass the time*
- *Reassure your partner if she's feeling afraid*
- *Encourage her to rest if she's buzzing with excitement*
- *Stay well fed and hydrated*
- *Monitor contractions to spot a pattern, but don't get obsessed*

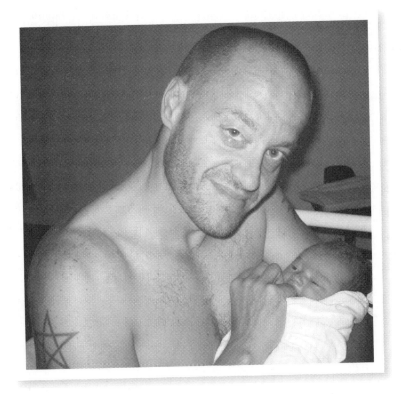

ADAM SPENCER'S STORY

You will never be served better and faster in a café than when you tell them your wife is in the early stages of labour.

Adam Spencer has a dicky eye as the result of a forceps delivery by an inexperienced doctor in 1969. With a great face for radio, a first class honours degree in pure mathematics and razor-sharp wit, he began his broadcasting career in 1996 when he won the Triple J Raw Comedy Championship. After some casual presenting on the Js, he took over the breakfast timeslot, presenting with Wil Anderson for six years. During this time he was also presenting ABC TV's Quantum and FAQ programs, shows that allowed him to indulge in his passion for science. Adam has been a regular guest on TV's Good News Week, The Fat and The Glasshouse among other TV hosting gigs. He has toured nationally with his shows The Last Time Tour (with Wil Anderson) and The Sleek Geek Tour (with Dr Karl). In his spare time, Adam coaches the University of Sydney's second grade women's soccer team. But there's also a serious side to Mr Spencer. He has served on the Senate of the University of Sydney, the NSW Premier's Advisory Committee on Greenhouse and Global Warming and the NSW Health Department's Clinical Ethics Review Committee, as well as being a supporter of the Fred Hollows Foundation, among other charities. Adam has reached the grand finals of the World Universities Debating Championship three times and was once crowned Best Speaker in the World. He's never been at a loss for words, but the births of his daughters left him gobsmacked.

I met my wife Mel at the Clock Hotel in Surry Hills on 28 February 2003. I saw the most beautiful woman I have ever seen walk in and sit down with her boyfriend. It was trivia night so my game plan was to help her with her answers. The first words I ever said to my wife were, 'The actor is George Clooney and the film is Solaris.' The boyfriend turned out to be just a good friend so when he left, I went in for the kill, pulling answers out of my arse like nobody's business.

A couple of years later, when Mel fell pregnant, it was a tremendous surprise for us. I was stunned more than anything. For reasons that are none of anyone's business, we'd assumed we couldn't fall pregnant at all, so having decided that Mel was the one for me, I had become at ease with the idea that I might never have children. I like to think that I redefined fertility in our case. I was in Brisbane doing a show and when I came off air, there were about 17 missed messages from Mel with the stunning news.

When she was 26 weeks pregnant, an ultrasound suggested things might already be starting to give, well before they should have and there was a chance that Mel could have the baby dangerously early. For the next seven weeks she was on doctor's orders of total bed rest. We moved the mattress from upstairs to downstairs and she only left that mattress to visit a doctor or go to the toilet. Once I came home and caught her at the fridge and she was in big trouble. At 33 weeks we were given the OK that she could go into labour anytime after that.

Ironically, when Mel was in labour we had to work pretty hard to get Ellie out and they had to break her waters to make it happen!

Mel went into labour not long after my last day on air, after which I was having a year off from breakfast radio. We couldn't have picked better timing. There was no more getting up at 3.20am for me so I was sleeping in like a *machine*. I woke up at 8am and Mel was tidying up in a primeval nesting kind of way and I thought, 'She's going to have this baby today.'

She'd been having contractions for a couple of hours but it was all under control so we went out for breakfast. You will never be served better and faster in a café than when you tell them your wife is in the early stages of labour.

The entire labour was about 12 hours and we stayed at home as long as we could. Once contractions got serious, we went into Royal Prince Alfred Hospital. The midwife there was an absolutely superb woman and it all went very smoothly.

I was in charge of the gas. The only time I felt a bit scared was when I forgot to hand the gas to Mel and she turned to me and screamed, 'GAS!' That kept me on my toes and reminded me that we still had a long way to go on this particular performance.

If you asked Mel, she would say that I had been given a limited set of duties and that I performed them acceptably. We clicked as a team but not in a 50/50 kind of way. I can't take any credit for the work that Mel did to give birth. However, I was there when she needed me and when she needed me to piss off and give her some space, I did that well.

Three hours after we arrived at the hospital, Ellie was born. Hers was a suction birth and just after she was born I was thinking, 'Am I the only one who realises that she has a really bad shape to her head?' She had blood on her head and it looked like her brain was leaking out! I was just about to say something when I realised that the shape to her head was exactly the same size and shape as the suction cup. Glad I chose not to speak.

Ellie's birth was ridiculously well timed in the scheme of things. Mel was a full time mother and I could be home about 75% of the time so I threw myself into fatherhood like no one's business, which I just loved doing. It was like we had the world's best ever parental leave conditions thrust upon us.

I'd done breakfast radio for so long that I was used to the kind of sleep routine you can expect from a newborn. Up at 3.20am.

We both really wanted a second child and Mel wanted to avoid another summer pregnancy so we had one 'preseason hit out' before

Mel's birthday. The next time I solicited another 'preseason hit out', Mel was feeling unwell and it transpired that she was already pregnant.

I like to boast that we really only tried to have a baby once but we have conceived twice. I like to think that there are subtle and complex ways that two people combine for maximum fertility. I feel so lucky that we didn't have fertility problems.

The week before Olivia was born, I had said on air that if I didn't show up for work one day, it would mean that our baby had been born. At about 2am on the Friday morning of that week (what was meant to be my last day on air for the year), Mel woke me to say she was in labour so I called someone in to cover my shift and we waited for the contractions to quicken. It turned out to be a substantial false labour, but by this time my shift had finished. The specialist said that he'd induce labour the next day.

I was like a kid who knew he was getting a BMX the next day, I just didn't know what colour. I was so excited.

That night I went to a cocktail reception at Sydney University and due to my on-air absence that morning, a lot of people assumed we'd had the baby. They were all congratulating me on the birth. I couldn't believe they thought I'd be out at a cocktail reception.

Olivia's birth was challenging. Basically, she wouldn't engage and after several hours Mel was getting very tired. The specialist had to take a very aggressive course of action – not for publication – to get Olivia out.

It was a December birth and I think we had a resident doctor who had only been out of uni for a couple of weeks. When the specialist did what he had to do to get the baby out, I looked at this poor pimply-faced resident turning white as a sheet as he was backing out of the room. We may have destroyed his medical career.

Mel was a gymnast in her youth. Once, she injured herself in a tumble run demonstration on a concrete floor but finished the routine on a broken foot. Not only does she have immense pain tolerance, she has impressive mental strength.

During the births Mel was remarkably calm even though she was in great discomfort while she was expending great amounts of energy. If I could have, I would have given birth to Olivia myself, not that I could have handled it like Mel. I'm almost jealous that I'll never know how it feels to give birth.

Ellie came in to meet her sister but the enclosed space of a hospital room is not an ideal place for a two-and-a-half year old so I took her for a walk on the Sydney Uni cricket fields. I was talking to one of the cricketers when Ellie just took off, running full speed. I'd never seen her do that before. It was such a beautiful moment to see my eldest child do something I had never seen her do before, just a couple of hours after my second child was born.

After things had settled I went to the shops in Newtown to get some supplies for our hospital stay. I hadn't eaten all day so I bought a chicken kebab on King Street. It was twilight on a beautiful summer's day, I was walking back towards the hospital and I bit into that kebab – I remember it so clearly – and it was the nicest meal I have had in my whole life. It tasted SO GOOD. I was just so happy with everything in the world.

Breakfast radio really is the perfect gig when you've got young kids. I'm up at 3.20am every morning so I don't see the girls before work but then I'm home by midday so I can pick Ellie up from school and spend time with both my girls. We have them in bed by 7.30pm and then I say, 'Daddy needs bottle and bed too,' and I'm off to bed shortly after them.

We couldn't be happier with two such gorgeous girls. I'm a bit of a greenie and while I don't judge those who have seven or eight offspring, in good conscience, I couldn't do it.

With more than two children you've moved from man-on-man defence to the floating defence zone. You've permanently got one in the sin bin and you're trying to cover that person in defence. We're quite fine with two children, thanks.

I try to not be in anyway prescriptive or evangelical when it comes to fatherhood. All I can say is that we're very, very lucky.

CHAPTER 9

FIRST STAGE OF LABOUR

The first stage of labour is a busy one. The cervix dilates and the uterus is working hard. Initially, the pain will seem manageable but as it ramps up your partner will not be speaking during contractions. She may still have her sense of humour between contractions but as dilation progresses, she will need her entire attention (and yours) focused on every contraction.

Now is the time to turn your phone off. You will live, I promise. Don't be making or accepting calls or sending and receiving texts or emails. You need to stay focused on your partner and she doesn't want you reporting on her progress to anyone. Work will have to wait. Even if you're the IT guy at the Australian Stock Exchange. I just made that up – I'm not referring to anyone in particular!

As it progresses, the first stage of labour can be the most physically tiring part of the birth for you as a support person, especially if your partner is labouring naturally. You'll both be working hard.

Establish and maintain your pain management routine and remember not to speak during contractions. As the pain ramps up, add things to the pain management mix such as essential oils or an extra heat pack, but add them slowly. Don't pull out the full box and dice at the start. Refer to your pain management arsenal to see what's next on your list if your partner is not coping with the pain. Help her to establish a positive *ahhhhh* sound as she uses her voice to give you an audible bell curve of her contraction.

Offer water between contractions – don't wait for her to ask for a drink. Once your partner is thirsty, she's already on the way to becoming dehydrated. Use a bendy straw to make it easy to offer her fluids even if she's lying down or on all fours. She'll be breathing through her mouth so her lips will become dry and she'll also need some lip balm.

Women in labour usually want heat on their bodies to help manage the pain. This means that her face gets hot and bothered and she needs to cool it down. Offer her a cold, wet washcloth for her forehead and ice cubes to suck on if you're using heat to manage the pain.

At some point during the first stage of labour you will need to make the move from home to hospital. I am often asked when the best time for that would be. This really depends on your partner. Some women don't feel safe and secure until they have arrived at the hospital. Then they can relax and focus on giving birth. Others feel safer at home and want to go to hospital just for the last few hours of labour.

Communicate with your caregivers about your partner's progress and they will tell you when it is time to come in. They will probably be keen to have you in the birthing unit as soon as labour is established.

When I gave birth to our first child, we didn't contact the hospital until contractions were about two minutes apart and lasting over a minute. The pain had been quite manageable and I was happy at home and wanted to stay there for as long as I could. Bruce called the hospital once I thought I was ready to go and I could hear the midwife exclaiming, 'GET HER IN HERE, QUICK!' Leaving it until contractions were two minutes apart was leaving it quite late. In the end, it was another five hours before our baby was born so it wasn't a big deal, but that might not necessarily have been the case.

Subsequent births are usually faster than first births though, so if your partner is birthing for the second or third time, get in there quick smart! For your second baby, once contractions are consistently lasting 60 seconds, regardless of how far apart they are, you should be on your way to hospital.

For your first birth, don't make the mistake of bolting off to hospital too early. If your partner's labour is not established, you will probably be sent back home, which is really demoralising, not to mention tiring. I know a woman who had 13 hours of prelabour, which she thought had progressed into established labour, so her husband took her to hospital. She was not dilating yet so she was sent home. She delivered her baby three weeks later!

Once you've made the decision to make the move to hospital, you should know the best route at any time of day. Plan this ahead of time. Which way will you go during peak hour? Which way would be best at 3am? You need to get your partner there safely, not quickly. The cops won't give you a police escort, they'll give you a speeding ticket, so play it safe and get your partner there within the speed limit.

The length of time you have to spend in the car should also factor into your decision regarding when to leave home. Some people choose to birth at hospitals that are a long way from home so a plan for this is important. While you are driving your partner to hospital, you can't be helping her with her pain management routine and she will not be comfortable.

If you have an hour's drive ahead of you (yes, a lot of people will drive past two or three maternity hospitals to get to the hospital they will be birthing at) consider leaving home before the stage where your partner cannot speak during contractions. It would be no picnic for her to spend an hour sitting in a car with a seat belt on in the throes of full-on labour and you'd be helpless to support her with anything other than verbal reassurances.

Make sure you know where the night entrance is for the labour ward or birth unit. The main doors to the hospital are locked at night so there is another door for maternity patient arrivals. In small hospitals this will probably be via the emergency department but in larger hospitals it will be somewhere else. Don't make your partner labour in the car park while you figure it out. Go to the hospital beforehand and find this entrance. You will probably be shown where it is when you do a tour during hospital-based antenatal classes.

There was a case at a hospital on the Central Coast of New South Wales a few years ago where a couple arrived at the main doors of the hospital at midnight. He was a rough-looking chap with tatts covering both arms and when he realised that they were locked out he just pounded on the front doors shouting and swearing. Understandably, the staff called security, but by the time they arrived, Tatt Man's partner had had her baby in the car.

The moral to that story is, know where the night entrance is for the maternity unit.

For some women, the change from home to hospital causes their labour to stall. This is the adrenal gland messing with the hormonal progress of childbirth. Just the new surroundings may make your partner feel anxious because she's in, what can feel for her, like a weak or compromised condition. She'll also be accepting a midwife into the support team and if this isn't a smooth transition, your partner may feel a little anxious or annoyed. This will produce adrenalin and as you know, this will block the all-important hormones that drive the labour and mask the pain.

So, get moving! Establish the birthing environment and make your partner feel comfortable. Do the following as soon as you arrive in your birth suite:

- Unpack your things so that you know where everything is. You shouldn't be constantly asking your partner, 'Where's the massage oil? Where's the iPod? What did I do with the camera?'
- Set up your music and hit play.
- Kill the lights and draw the blinds. The best combination for lighting is the room light off and the bathroom light on. That gives your caregivers enough light to see what they're doing but lets your

partner labour in low light.

- Once your partner is comfortable, make another trip to the car if you need to collect more things or to move your car into longer term parking if you're in emergency parking.
- Meet and greet your midwife, remember her name and start using it.
- Familiarise yourself with all the resources in the room. Open all the drawers and cupboards and see what's where, including extra towels, blankets, pillows and washcloths.
- Find the vomit bags and put one by the bed. If they're needed, it'll be in a hurry and you won't have time to hunt them down.
- Ask for a large jug of water with ice cubes if you don't have one in the room already.
- Find out where the ice machine is and the coffee and tea facilities while you're at it.

Once all this is done, relax, sit quietly and let the room be calm and quiet, then re-establish the pain management routine that you had going at home. Enjoy the stillness between contractions. Kiss her and tell her you love her.

On arrival, your partner will have her basic observations done by a midwife: pulse, blood pressure, temperature as well as a check on the baby's heart beat with a doppler. Some hospitals routinely monitor the labouring woman for the first 30 minutes after arrival with a foetal monitor that also tracks contractions.

This is a good time to mention your birth plan to the midwife. Just give it to her verbally, in a nutshell. For example, 'We'd like to try for a natural birth so please don't offer drugs unless we ask,' or 'We're keen on an epidural so can you call the anaesthetist?' Let the midwife know about anything out of the ordinary such as signs of green discharge if that should occur.

Keep that phone turned off! I once attended a birth for a barrister and his wife. He had a long trial commencing right before their due date so I was there partly because there was a good chance that he wouldn't make it to the birth. As it turned out, the baby was born during the night so he was able to be there but he wasn't exactly 'present'.

It was late at night and he was making calls to do with his trial in the loudest barrister voice I'd ever heard. I wanted to shout, 'OBJECTION! Your Honour, I would like to request that counsel for the plaintiff turn off the damn phone!' At one point he went into the bathroom – the most echo-prone room in the entire hospital – and shouted down the phone to his father, 'Yes! Dad! She's just having a vaginal exam!' His wife was horrified at the thought of her father-in-law being given this personal detail.

Once labour is cranking along and she's dilated beyond five centimetres, you will need to be fully present, give her your full attention and participate in every contraction. Being fully present doesn't just mean being in the room.

I remember a woman whose husband was an IT boffin. By the end of the birth, he had read the entire operations manual for the foetal monitor and could show the midwives how to change the paper roll in the machine. However, his partner said that he hadn't really been focused on her and she felt alone and unsupported. Try not to get distracted by the fascinating medical side of it all. Stay focused on your partner and each contraction.

At another birth I attended, the woman was having a VBAC or vaginal birth after Caesarean. This usually requires foetal monitoring for the entire labour so she was attached to a foetal monitor. While she laboured away, her husband, her obstetrician, the midwife and the anaesthetist stood in a neat little semicircle around the monitor, chit-chatting while they ignored the birthing woman. After the birth she said to me, 'You were the only person in the room who was actually there for me.' It wasn't as if the baby's heartbeat was fluctuating – it sat steadily on 135 beats per minute – but that was where their focus was. Make

How long will labour last?

Ha! The 64 Million Dollar Question. The average first labour lasts 12 to 18 hours. Some first labours are shorter and some are longer. The length of labour only accounts for active labouring and doesn't include prelabour. This means she could have, for example, a 12 hour prelabour, followed by a 17 hour active labour and be within the average length of time for a first labour. Go to hospital prepared for a 24 hour slog so that you will be well equipped. Don't focus on the time during the labour. You are on birth time.

sure that *you* are the person who is in the room just for your partner.

Stick with your pain management routine if it is working for your partner, only changing or adding something to the mix if she needs it or if the routine stops working for her. Make sure that you both stay hydrated through this stage – usually the longest stage of labour.

Encourage her to sleep if she has an epidural. Some women get very chatty once the epidural kicks in but often the whole point of an epidural is to allow the woman some rest so she can push her baby out naturally. Turn off all the lights, tell the staff that you're sleeping, and have a snooze – probably the last nap you'll get for a while.

For those who experience a stall in labour or a labour that is progressing very slowly, there are a number of things you can try to help kick things off again and fend off the augmentation of labour by means of a Syntocinon drip which will produce very painful contractions.

Firstly, take her to the bathroom. Labour can stall if she has a full bladder. You're doing the right thing by giving her lots of fluids but she may need prompting to go to the toilet.

Make sure she is nice and warm. Hospitals can be very cold and your partner may be dressed to suit the temperature in your house rather than the hospital. Put some warm socks on her feet and give her a blanket. If she is really cold, you can request blankets that are warmed in a blanket heater. A warm shower will warm her up too and will keep gravity working to bring your baby down. Avoid the bath when labour has stalled. A hot bath is your pain management 'big gun' that you want to save for when the going gets tough.

Go for a little walk up the hall, keep your conversation focused on her, the birth and your baby. Don't think that talking about other things will help distract her from the stalled birth. She needs to stay in the primal brain to birth. Keep your language positive and gentle.

Ask your partner if there is anything bothering her. It might be you who's bothering her, so be prepared for that and do whatever you have to, to help her be calm and relaxed. It may be a specific fear that she would like to talk about. Let her voice her fear and then assure her that she's in good hands and that you're with her in this.

She may just want to vent about something. She might be cross with her mother for trying to muscle in on the birth or something else that wouldn't necessarily occur to you. Let her have a vent, validate her feelings and then give her a nice back and shoulder rub.

Men are really good at fixing things, but this situation is one thing you just can't fix. You have to go with the flow, love your partner, be gentle with her and wait for labour to kick off again.

Some women go right through labour without any internal vaginal exams, others have one when they get to hospital in labour and another before they actively start pushing. Vaginal exams are not pleasant. Your partner has to lie on her back to allow the obstetrician or midwife to assess dilation accurately and any contractions she has in this position are more painful and harder to manage. Her caregivers can do a vaginal exam if your partner is in any position, but it is easier to get a more accurate interpretation if she's on her back.

The results of vaginal exams can be demoralising. If your partner is told that she's three centimetres dilated when she's been in labour all day and was hoping for seven or eight centimetres, she will be disappointed in her progress and may feel that she can't continue. On the other hand, if you're told that she's eight centimetres dilated, this can be very encouraging.

My colleague Jane said that this was true for her. She was induced and after four or five hours of very intense labour, her midwife assured her that she'd be at least seven centimetres dilated. A vaginal exam revealed that she was between one and two centimetres dilated and Jane said she just wanted to cry.

It's important to note that the cervix does not dilate at the same rate throughout labour. It can take 12 hours to get to six centimetres and then only a couple of hours to go from six to ten. A woman can take a whole day to get to nine centimetres and only half an hour to get from there to fully dilated. Five centimetres therefore does not represent the half way mark. Frustrating, I know. You can't use dilation as a progress indicator any more than you can say the half time score is an indicator of who's going to win the match.

Stage one of labour is really the lion's share of the work when it comes to childbirth support so make sure you remember these points:

- *Make the move from home to hospital safely*
- *As soon as you arrive at the hospital, establish your birthing environment and get settled*
- *Be fully present for your partner (not just in the room)*
- *Establish and maintain a pain management routine*
- *Keep yourself and your partner well hydrated*
- *If labour stalls: keep her warm, make sure she empties her bladder, let her vent her concerns if she needs to*

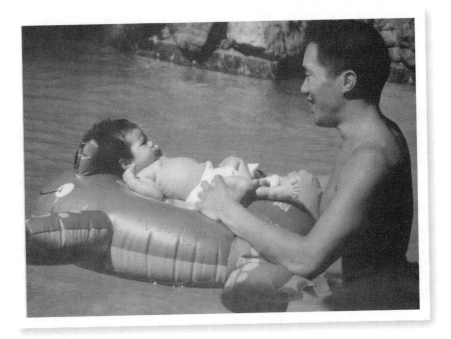

CHARLIE TEO'S STORY

Dr Charlie Teo is a neurosurgeon specialising in paediatrics. After twelve years of education and specialist training, Charlie and his wife Genevieve, a nurse, left Australia for a 10-year stint in the US where they had three of their four daughters. When their eldest child came home from school after 'gunshot drill training' they decided it was time to head home to Australia. Charlie is a director of the Centre for Minimally Invasive Neurosurgery and a founding director of the Cure for Life Foundation, an organisation funding research into treatment for brain cancer, the number one cancer killer in children. He is a pioneer in neuro-endoscopy techniques and continues to train surgeons all over the world. Charlie has copped criticism from some of his peers for breaking with the conservative image of neurosurgeons by playing the bagpipes, riding a motorcycle, wearing Hawaiian shirts and for courting the media. For the record, it took three months of asking before he agreed to the interview for this book. On the other hand, Charlie is wholeheartedly adored by his patients, many of whom have little hope until Dr Teo is willing to operate. He spends four months a year giving his services to patients in developing countries and has been nominated for the Australian of the Year Award many times. He believes that childbirth is the most natural event on earth that shouldn't be interfered with or coached. He also found the change in the status quo after the birth of his first child to be quite a shock.

We hadn't planned on having a large family; in fact I had been quite vocal that I would only ever have two children in order to be socially and environmentally responsible. I felt it was irresponsible from a population viewpoint to have lots of kids. However, I just loved having children so much and I really wanted a boy so I kept thinking we would have just one more shot at a son. By the time we had three girls – I just loved having three kids as opposed to two – I thought, bugger it, let's try one more time – and she's a girl too! There's no difference really between having three and four kids, in fact four is a little easier because your eldest can help to nurture the fourth child.

I was a bad boy when I was young, a bit of a womaniser. I never treated women badly, I have great respect for women, but I had a lot of girlfriends. I think having four daughters was my due return.

Our first baby was born in the States. I thought I would do what I was expected to do, that is, be the nurturing, caring husband. I went to the antenatal classes, but was kicked out after the first one. I'm a bit of a philistine and I'm not into all that touchy-feely sort of stuff. There were all these breathing exercises and I thought it was all pretty humorous and laughed. Genevieve said, 'Fine, don't come back again!'

When we got to the birth I decided that all that coached breathing is crap! Birth is such a natural phenomena, I think it's wrong to try to teach someone what comes naturally.

When I went through med school, we had a year of tutoring in 'personality': interviewing skills, empathy, warmth and compassion. I don't think you can teach that. We'd have to do role-plays and they would try to teach us the best verbal response to a patient. I'd sit back from these tutorials and think, 'That poor bastard over there has no social skills whatsoever and here he is repeating these sentences like a robot.'

I thought childbirth was the same. Here they were trying to teach Genevieve to do something that should come naturally to her. They were also trying to tell me how to behave and respond to things in just the right way and I thought that was unnatural. I didn't go to any more antenatal classes and I'm so glad she let me off the hook.

Being Mr Au Naturel, I didn't want Genevieve to have an epidural or anything unnatural. I couldn't appreciate the pain that women go through or the joys of modern medicine in the field of obstetrics but I wanted her to give birth naturally and she respected that and went all natural for about 12 hours. She eventually had an epidural. Genevieve doesn't regret having an epidural, but she held it against me for making her hold off for so long.

Genevieve was quite abusive to me in labour! I remember lying in bed with her trying to be Mr Touchy Feely and rubbing her back when she snapped, 'You smell!' I'd been sitting there for twelve hours so maybe I did. I just sucked it up, tolerated the abuse and did my best. 'Don't touch me!' she said at one point.

After she had the epidural I played the doctor role rather than the father role and I'm glad I did. She became hypotensive after the epidural and her blood pressure dropped to something like 50 on 20, which is very low. You're meant to give fluids when this happens and there was no one around so I pumped the fluids into her. After that I felt like I had a purpose and I was needed. I'd done my bit so that was good.

When the baby was coming out, I didn't go down that end. As a medical student I had seen how unattractive it looks. You've got this huge big vagina staring at you, with the head coming out and fluid everywhere. The mother is red and sweaty. It's just an ugly sight and I didn't want to see that with my wife. So I stayed up the top end.

The obstetrician tried to get me to play the father role again and have me cut the cord but I didn't want to, as I saw that as her job. There's this dictum in medicine that says that if you operate on or deal with a doctor or a doctor's family, things are going to go wrong. I think that's because you might treat a doctor a little differently as a patient and not do what you would normally do. So I wanted to make it very clear to that doctor that I didn't want her to do anything differently from her usual routine.

When I operate on doctors and their families, I appreciate it when they don't try to be a doctor. I need to treat them like a layperson and talk to them like a layperson, like I treat everyone else. I'm pleased to say that by adopting that philosophy with my own doctor-patients, I haven't had the misfortune of having many complications with those patients.

Then the baby came and it was a great moment. Suddenly Genevieve's nasty streak turned nice and she was smiley and happy! She was like Jekyll and Hyde. She'd been yelling and swearing at me and now she was all smiles.

At one point I had tried to use a little of the breathing technique I remembered from that one and only class and she said, 'Just get lost! I can't do it!' That confirmed for me that those eight weeks of breathing classes were a total waste of time.

I recall being pleased when the placenta came out because I know what happens if the placenta is retained. Delivery of the placenta was like an afterthought or anticlimax really. From a medical point of view I was pleased when that happened and I was watching out for it but from an emotional father's point of view it didn't mean anything.

Alex was a delightful baby. I was born to be a father. I have always loved kids, which is why I did paediatric neurosurgery. I can remember when I was a young fella preferring to play with kids and little babies rather than playing macho games. I knew I would love my own kids.

Becoming a father completely changed my response to my patients and their families. It's just terrible when I treat a child exactly the same age as my own, with the same little expressions and attitude. It's very hard to separate the emotion from the science of it all.

By the time Nikky, our second, was born, I considered myself a bit of a veteran in the childbirth stakes. I was doing my ward rounds and thought I would just wait until the time arrived and Genevieve needed me. Again, I wasn't too touchy-feely and wasn't too supportive of Genevieve, nor did she demand it, although she was a little embarrassed by the fact that she couldn't say that her husband was by her side. I think I was even operating while she was in labour and they called me when they said she was about to deliver. I was a fellow then, not the main surgeon, so I broke off from the operating room and went to be with her.

For our third daughter, I sat with Genevieve the whole time because she had been a bit upset about my absence for most of the second birth. But I was on the phone to Italy a lot, organising a neurosurgery conference and after a while she said, 'Go then, go! You're no help – just get out!' So I did get out of there and I came back for the important part at the end.

All the expats in Little Rock, Arkansas stuck together and Genevieve's friend, another expat, was in labour at exactly the same time so they kept each other company.

The last labour was very quick with no time for an epidural, funny gas or any intervention at all. Just two contractions and the baby popped out.

I wanted to write a book after our second child was born, so guys could read about what to expect at this time in their lives. I wanted to tell guys that they have got to expect to have no attention from their partner, before, during and after the birth. There's no sex, nurturing or pampering from your partner.

Men are real wusses, they're like babies and you need to pamper them, care for them and stroke their ego. Then a baby comes along and you take second place. So as a father you have to somehow get it in your mind that this is the natural process. You have to stop putting yourself as number one, stop getting upset about it and not seek the attention from somewhere else.

Guys need sex, several times a week. We just need it. It's not just sex though, it's intimacy and attention from your partner. You don't get any of that when a baby comes along. It would have helped me to know what I was in for and that others had been through it before me. Had I known that there was a light at the end of the tunnel, that this wasn't permanent, it would have been easier for me to adjust.

I wish I had known to expect 'pregnant brain syndrome' where women just can't think the way they used to. It's caused by sleep deprivation as well as a micro-embolism caused by the birth. This is a documented neurological outcome where something such as air, placental juices, fats or blood clots can get into the blood system and lodge in the brain to form a microinfarct or mini stroke. It's a real, physiological, neurological syndrome. Husbands need to be warned that their wife won't be thinking straight. She'll be very emotional and guys just have to suck it up, expect it and get on with it.

I believe that you have to train your children or modify their behaviour so that they are pleasant little people to be with and you enjoy their company. Genevieve and I have different standards when it comes to behaviour. For example, I let them swear because I swear like a trooper, but Genevieve doesn't tolerate it. This isn't a source of acrimony between us; the kids know our individual limits.

When I have time off from work I just crave to be with my children and so does Genevieve. I can't wait to be with them. We have four beautiful daughters and I love them very much.

CHAPTER 10

TRANSITION – DUCK FOR COVER!

Transition is at the very end of the first stage of labour when the baby's head comes right down into the pelvis and your partner dilates the last couple of centimetres. This is when labour pain hits its peak and it is a very common time for women to throw any plans for a natural birth out the window and ask for drugs.

I did! By this stage of my first birth I had had enough and I asked my midwife, 'What are my pain relief options here?' She just brushed me off, saying, 'Oh come on, you're about to have your baby! Not long now,' and she walked out of the room. This actually gave me a bit of a second wind – sometimes it's easy to forget that you're having a baby. You can get so wound up with the birth process that you forget about the prize at the end.

'Women going through transition can be wide-eyed and wild,' says Hannah Dahlsen who's seen her fair share of women in labour as a midwife of twenty years. 'There is a massive surge of hormones, an avalanche that rushes through the body during transition. Some women start grasping at things, others shout at their husband, cursing and swearing, or declare that they have had enough. We don't understand transition well enough nor do we really know the great variation with which women respond to the rush of hormones during this fascinating stage of labour.'

Hannah believes that from an evolutionary perspective, this is the cave woman's need to be safe, to get some attention and be protected. Your job is to validate these feelings and make her feel safe.

Bruce had his hands full when I rocketed through transition during our son's birth. I was grumpy and too exhausted to actively participate in my pain management routine. Bruce kept his cool and massaged my back furiously. I couldn't let him leave my side for a second.

Transition is often when there is a significant change in a woman's mood. Things might have been working well, your pain management routine may have worked well for hours and then suddenly it stops working for her and she doesn't know where to put her hands or can't get comfortable.

In transition, some women suddenly say that they are afraid. They may have laboured calmly and confidently and then they're suddenly crying and telling you that they're not coping.

If she is going to lose the plot, it will be during transition, when the pain is at its worst. Some women report just wanting to give up. They want to leave this birthing caper to someone else. Some women even visualise themselves walking out of the room. I remember looking at my doula and saying, 'Can you do this for me for a little while so I can have a nap?'

This would be a very bad time to suggest that your partner 'relax'. She can't relax at the peak of labour and you deserve to be clobbered if you suggest it.

If the mood changes and things stop working for your partner, change the scene. Get her out of the shower, dry her off and help her into a comfortable position on the bed. Put some socks on her feet and throw a sheet over her. Or, if she hasn't had a bath or a shower yet, this is the perfect time to make that move.

Transition can be very intense and challenging if you and your partner are already tired. Take charge if she panics and tells you that she is afraid. Assure her that she's getting there and is doing well. Ask her what she's afraid of. Often it's something that she can be easily reassured about. If she says she's afraid of the pain you can tell her that this is as bad as it gets, that she's managing and it won't go on forever.

Lots of women say, 'I can't do this!' and the best thing to say is, 'But you already are, you're doing it right now and you're doing it perfectly. You've come so far and I'm so proud of you. Just get through the next contraction.'

Just after transition, some women experience what Hannah describes as a lull, where contractions slow right down and women can take a little rest before the hard work of pushing begins. In a homebirth environment, the midwife might tuck the woman into bed for a snooze during this stage. In hospitals, caregivers are more likely to put in a drip to augment the labour and keep it cranking. Ask your caregivers if there is a medical necessity for this and submit to some extra foetal monitoring if that will give your partner the freedom to ride out this period without drugs to influence the progress of labour.

If she has the urge to push, tell your midwife. Your caregivers will probably want to check that your partner is ten centimetres dilated before she starts to actively push. Her *ahhhhhhing* may turn into little involuntary grunts, which is a good sign too. If she starts to make these sounds, mention it to your caregivers and they'll start busying themselves with delivery trolleys and at this point, if you're in private care, they'll probably let your obstetrician know when it would be time to come in.

Your partner may say she wants to do a poo, which usually just means she's ready to deliver her baby. The baby's head borrows space from the bowel so pushing a baby out really does feel like doing the world's biggest dump. I expected birthing a baby to feel vaginal but it doesn't. It feels anal. There you have it.

This is why some babies born to women who have no professional care when they are in labour are born into the toilet. It's OK for her to sit on the toilet for a little while. First babies generally don't come out like rockets. However, if she says she has the urge to push, move her onto the bed or a mattress on the floor and help her into a comfortable position for pushing.

I remember being at a birth where the obstetrician wore huge, white rubber gumboots like a worker at the fish markets, obviously quite a character, which sort of explains this next story. He was sitting on a stool right there in front of the birthing mother's vagina as she started to make some involuntary grunts or pushes. Suddenly, she did a massive trumpeting fart in the obstetrician's face. She shot a look of horror and embarrassment at me, but the doctor was thrilled. 'Fantastic!' he said. 'More room for the baby! Can you do me another one?'

If she farts, she'll probably be embarrassed. Don't tease her – she's in no mood to be gracious.

Your partner may do a poo as the baby's head pushes down and leans on the bowel – and your job is not to make a fuss of it. Just whip it away and flush it down the loo. Scoop it out of the bath, wash it down the drain in the shower – whatever you have to do to deal with it quickly. No one likes to poo with an audience so just deal with it with minimal fuss. Remember the negative effects of adrenalin and make sure your partner is not embarrassed or annoyed that she's had to empty her bowels.

I was at a birth where the birthing mother just happened to have full bowels and for about half an hour, as the baby's head came down through the birth canal, she gradually emptied her bowels. She hated it and after a while shouted at no one in particular, 'I just keep shitting!'

The best thing to do if she's having to poo is to hunt down the 'blueys': large rectangular absorbent sheets with a blue plastic backing. All hospitals have them and there should be a stash in your room. Put one of these under your partner to catch the mess and whip it away when it needs replacing.

Enough said about bowel motions in labour?

Transition can last anywhere from five minutes to half an hour or longer. It may pass you by without you noticing a significant change in your partner, or it may be the most challenging part of the entire birth.

If you hadn't even heard of transition until now, review the following points to remember:

- *Transition is when the pain is at its absolute peak – stay close*
- *If your partner loses the plot, take charge and reassure her*
- *If your pain management routine stops working for her, change the scene*
- *If she starts to grunt, let your caregivers know*
- *If she needs to poo, deal with it*

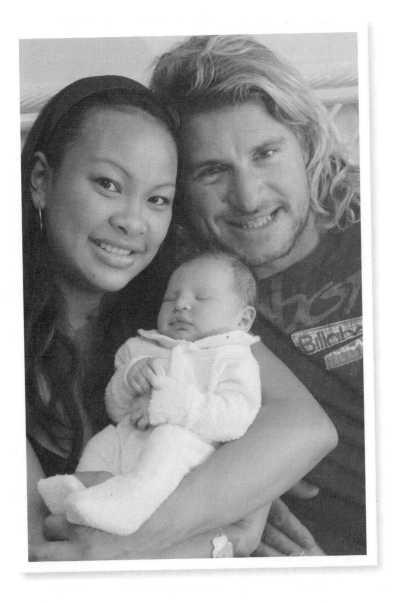

MARK OCCHILUPO'S STORY

I was so happy – even happier than when I won the world title!

Mark Occhilupo first learned to surf at Kurnell in Sydney's south when he was only six or seven years old, on an old surf board that had been left out for council clean up. By the age of 13 the goofy footer had surfboard and wetsuit sponsors and by 14 had reached the finals in the Pro-Am competition. By 17, Mark had dropped out of school and passed selection for the professional surf tour on his very first attempt. For the next five years he remained in the top ten with only two other professional surfers at the time beating his winning percentages. He travelled the world on the Pro Tour, going back to Hawaii each winter to surf at Pipe so that he could come back to Australia super-fit and ready to compete on his home turf. In 1988, things took a dive and Occy suddenly quit the professional surfing circuit, disillusioned with the Pro Tour, never having won the world champion title that many thought he deserved. He spent the next decade fighting obesity, depression and a total lack of motivation, a time that he refers to as his 'Elvis years'. In 1997 at the ripe old age of 30, when most professional surfers have already surfed their better years, Occy requalified for the World Championship Tour, finishing second in the world during his first year back on tour. Then, in 1999 at the age of 33, with most of the competitors about half his age, Occy stunned the world by winning the world champion title. For the next eight years, he remained in the world's top 20, eventually retiring in 2007 at the age of 41. Occy is a fascinating character, a man everyone seems to have a soft spot for and whose kids think he's the best dad who ever lived.

I met my wife Mae not long after my first marriage ended. I'd had some wild single days for a while there but when I got together with Mae, she brought all that to an end.

Mae is a beautiful woman. She has a Filipino background with a large, extended family and we talked about having kids when we first got together. I hadn't been able to have kids with my first wife. I had been told that I had a low sperm count, but with Mae we didn't seem to have any problems and she fell pregnant like magic. I think it was because we were so in love. I was so happy – even happier than when I won the world title!

On the day our son was born, we still had about a month to go before the baby was due. It was a full moon and we were at home one evening with me watching the news and having a beer. Mae said she thought she was in labour and that we had better go to the hospital to have it checked out. We went into the hospital and they sent us home again, but we were back there again the same evening and Mae laboured through the night. She's not a big girl but she was so strong in there. The labour was about seven hours long and it was full on.

I did as much as I could to help Mae but I was nervous. She was strong though, so she made me feel strong. I can only imagine going through the process of childbirth.

Mae was kind of angry with me at one point because between contractions she saw me having a go on the happy gas, just to calm my nerves. She wasn't too happy with that. I haven't been on that stuff since I was at the dentist when I was a kid! But overall, Mae thinks I was pretty good helping her out through the labour. Let's just say that!

When it was time to push the baby out, I stayed up there with Mae to give her as much support as I could, holding her hand and cheering her on. She was using my fingers for grip and she squeezed them so tight that it was really painful.

Our baby boy came out and I cut the cord. When I first saw Jay and his little eyes opened, it was such a special moment. He gave me a worried little look as if to say, 'Will you be able to take care of me?' It was just so magic. I will never forget that first look between father and son, it was so vivid.

We named him Jay for two reasons. Firstly because it's my middle name and also because we're pretty sure he was conceived at Jeffreys Bay or J-Bay as we call it. That's a spot in South Africa that has the best waves.

Having a newborn at home was epic. Mae had set up the baby's room beautifully. Jay was such a bundle of joy and having him at home was so much fun but it was tiring. It was what I would call, ALL TIME.

After a few years we decided that we wanted another baby and conceiving Jonah was also like magic, no problems at all.

He came a few weeks early too, but his labour was much faster – only about three and a half hours. I was very useful during labour the second time as well! The midwives were great – we knew them all from our first baby's birth.

Both babies had some jaundice just after they were born. It was scary seeing my baby in the incubator – that freaked me out. The midwives said it was all pretty normal. They told me to sit with him in the sun to let him get some natural light to help treat the jaundice. I would unwrap the baby and hold him in my arms.

Mae is such a good mum. I travel a lot and so Mae does an awful lot of the parenting by herself. When I'm home, it's my turn. It's quite a workload with two kids.

We've worked out a good routine that works really well for us. I like to wake up really early in the morning and go for an early surf, then I come back home and help get the kids ready for school so that Mae can have a little sleep-in. I'm the Mum-Dad in the playground. Then I like to have an early night so I can be up in the surf again in the morning.

I took Jay out for his first surf at Sunset Beach in Hawaii, on a day when the waves were nice and small, which doesn't happen there often.

I took him out on a long board and paddled him out, a pretty special moment for a father and his son. We caught a wave and lay down together the whole way in. The look on his face was magic!

He's a pretty good little surfer and is in the under-sevens at Snapper Board Rider's Club. He's a good little skateboarder and snowboarder too. He's definitely got some talent.

Jonah's a great little kid. He comes along to Jay's rugby league matches and has his own little outfit on and thinks he's playing on the team. Jonah's just learning to swim so he's not surfing out the back yet. He surfs on his mini board in the lounge room at home, surfing down a mattress he has set up and when we go to the beach he stays in his wetsuit all day.

Mae and I took our little guys on the Pro Surfing Tour through Europe and South Africa. Jay was only about four and Jonah was one and those were the hardest trips I've ever done. The poor babies just wanted to get off the plane, but after one 12-hour flight we'd have another 12-hour flight to follow. It was full on.

I love being a dad and I'd love us to have another baby. We might see how we go…

CHAPTER 11

THE BIG PUSH AND THE MOMENT OF BIRTH

Pushing out a baby can be hard work. It can also be a lonely time for your partner because it's all up to her and you can't do the pushing for her.

'Second stage is approached in one of two ways,' says midwife Akal Khalsa who has been catching babies for over thirty years. 'Some midwives encourage the woman not to push until she has an overwhelming urge to do so. However, in most hospital labour wards, second stage will be actively managed, whereby your partner will be encouraged to push as soon as it has been determined that her cervix is fully dilated, but before she gets the urge.'

Some caregivers encourage women to 'breathe' their baby out. However, it often takes great maternal effort and a hell of a lot of pushing to deliver a baby through the birth canal for women birthing vaginally for the first time. Second and third babies might be breathed out, but first babies usually need pushing.

In most Australian hospitals, from the time a woman is fully dilated she has about two hours to push out her baby, before her medical caregivers will want to intervene and deliver the baby mechanically with forceps or by vacuum extraction. I am yet to meet a woman who wants a forceps delivery so you have your time cut out for you. Remember though, that you shouldn't put time pressure on your partner; this information is rather for you to keep in mind.

'One way to avoid the time pressure is to plan with your partner beforehand that when she starts to feel any pressure on her rectum, you keep it to yourselves for as long as possible,' suggests Akal. 'This will allow the baby to move into position before the labour ward staff start behaving like a cheer squad. In the homebirths I attend, I give the woman plenty of time for her body to become ready to push. Once she is overcome by the expulsive energy of the contraction, she is more likely to be able to breathe her baby out.'

I was at a birth where the couple wanted to breathe out their first baby but after 90 minutes of no progress, the midwife casually mentioned that we had 30 minutes to deliver the baby or there would be salad tongs involved. So that woman had to push incredibly hard to fend off any intervention. She managed it, but not without a spectacular tear as a result of such forceful pushing.

This can be quite a medically managed part of the birth with at least one midwife in attendance, the obstetrician and sometimes a paediatrician, if, for example, your baby was an IVF conception.

I'm always impressed that midwives seem to be so accurate at knowing when to call in the obstetrician for a woman in private care who is ready to birth her baby. The obstetrician always seems to arrive just in time. I asked midwife Hannah Dahlen how midwives manage to do this.

'Midwives are experienced in picking up on behavioural responses,' says Hannah. 'I can stand outside a room and listen to a woman and say, "she's seven centimetres". It's all about how she sounds, plus some visual indicators.'

During the pushing stage, the atmosphere can be quite different from the earlier part of labour, with people now shouting encouragement for your partner to PUSH!

Some women have an uncontrollable urge to push and there's just no way you can stop her when she's ready. Other women register little or no urge to push and need to consciously start pushing once they have been told that they're fully dilated.

When do I help my partner into the bath for a water birth?
According to Adelaide childbirth educator, doula and mother of seven, Helen Hriskin, the best time for a woman to immerse herself in the tub for a water birth is just before it is time to push. 'This allows a woman the freedom of movement she needs to actively manage labour before she starts the hard work of pushing,' says Helen who has given birth to two of her seven babies under water with husband Romeo and their other children by her side. 'I found the water soothing and supportive. There is also something about getting into a tub that makes me feel more comfortable with being naked,' says Helen. 'Water birth lets the guys off the hook when it comes to physically supporting their partner because the water handles the pain so effectively and carries much of the mother's weight.' If your partner is hoping to give birth in water, the hospital will need to be appropriately staffed for this. Each hospital has its own protocol on water birth, so talk to your caregivers well in advance. In the public hospital system, the midwife will need to be qualified to handle a water birth. If the midwife assigned to your partner's birth is not qualified, she won't allow your partner to start pushing in the bath and if your partner won't get out of the bath, the midwife will pull the plug! I've seen a birthing mother stand on the plug and demand a qualified midwife so that she could give birth in the water. Midwives in birth centres should all be water birth qualified, but in a regular public hospital labour ward you may find a midwife without these qualifications. Some birth suites have showers instead of baths while others have only shallow baths. If you birth at home you can hire a birth pool and install it in your living room.

Help your partner into a comfortable position for pushing. A birthing stool is good for pushing, but not for the crowning of the head and birth itself as it has a very high rate of contribution to tearing. To reduce the chance of a perineal tear, help your partner to position herself comfortably on all fours or on her side. These positions are better for keeping pressure off the perineum for the actual birth.

Your partner may be totally exhausted and will need you close by her side by the time she is fully dilated and ready to start pushing. Stay close by and whisper encouragement to her during contractions. Your words can override any negative medical talk in the room.

One of the first births I attended was with a lovely couple who had a straightforward first birth. When it was time to push out the baby, her obstetrician was in attendance. Boy, did he bellow at her while she was pushing. 'Puuuuuush! Puuuuuuush!' The baby came down the birth canal and we caught a glimpse of the head, but between contractions, the baby's head would slip back inside and out of sight. This is perfectly normal as the baby has to be pushed through the pubic arch. The obstetrician hollered at the birthing mother and then when the baby's head slipped out of sight between contractions, he'd say, 'Oh no, we've lost it again!'

This seemed so negative when her progress had been so good. Afterwards I asked the birthing mother if that had bothered her. She said, 'I didn't even know he was saying anything like that. All I could hear was your encouragement whispered in my ear.'

It is more painful to push so most women hold back when they first start to push with contractions. Encourage her to push through the pain and to bring your baby down. The technique for pushing is simple and you can help your partner get this right. My mum says she remembers this technique from when she first gave birth over 40 years ago and still uses it when she needs to open a tight lid on a jar! Not quite as challenging as pushing a baby through the birth canal but the same principle of holding the breath.

To push, your partner needs to take a huge breath, hold it and then push. Once she needs to take a breath, she should empty the lungs slowly, then take the next breath slowly. It's important that she doesn't rush filling the lungs again. This should be done slowly and calmly.

Try to include three giant pushes in every contraction. Then have a breather while she waits for the next contraction. Push with your partner until she gets this technique right. It takes most women about ten contractions before they get their groove and then they can push without much further guidance.

'Some women, in fact, find that the pain is more manageable when they start to push,' says Dr John Keogh. 'In a way they have been running from the pain and trying to keep it at bay for hours. Now they can turn around and attack it, take control of it and shake it by the scruff of the neck. It can help them to take control. It can be a very powerful experience.'

My brother Peter stood down the business end while his wife Kara was pushing out their little boy Luke. Pete gave her his loudest Lleyton Hewitt 'COME OOOOOON!' while she pushed. She told me later if he'd stood a bit closer, she'd have kicked him in the head.

You're not on the Fanatics' cheer squad, you're there to support your partner emotionally and physically. Use positive language and tell her when you can see the baby's head. Describe the baby's hair and help her reach down to touch it between contractions.

Some women have little naps between each contraction. Let her rest. Kiss your partner and tell her you love her. Thank her for doing this. She is doing you the biggest favour anyone has ever done or ever will, after your mother, who delivered you. Don't forget to give your mother a kiss later for going through this too!

You can offer a mirror so that your partner can see her progress as she's pushing. Some women thrive with this kind of visual reference so that they can see how hard they have to push to move the baby. Other women hate the thought of it and just want to push with their eyes shut.

Encourage your partner to relax her pelvic floor, to really open up and let go. Remember, you must never tell a woman in labour to 'relax'. She'll punch you. However, you can encourage her to relax a specific muscle. Remind her to relax her jaw. A lot of women clench their teeth when they're pushing and this is not ideal.

You may see a side of your partner that you have never seen before – a level of strength, determination and power that you may not have thought was possible, especially at the end of what might have been a long and exhausting journey. I'm warning you – you will look at your partner with a new sense of admiration and a kind of love you may not have experienced before. You will see her harness a type of primal strength that you didn't think possible and this may bring tears to your eyes. As a doula, I have seen this many, many times and it always makes me weepy. To witness a woman reach the end of a challenging journey in a position of strength and determination is amazing.

Seeing your baby emerge from your partner's body is one of the most miraculous things you'll ever witness. I recommend you have a look down the business end if you want to see the amazing sight. Some men say they find this quite disturbing and they'd rather not have a visual image of what their partner's vagina has been through. You decide.

Don't worry if your baby's head looks like something from outer space. This is very normal. The baby's head will probably be very wrinkly and compressed as it comes down the birth canal. And even if you are a family of blondes, your baby may be born with dark hair. Now would be a very bad time to question the paternity of the child. Many babies are born with fine dark hair that falls out in the first couple of months and is replaced with a blonde mop. My son was one of those.

When the baby's head crowns, just before the whole head pops out, your caregivers should encourage your partner to stop pushing. This will give the perineum much-needed time to stretch. Your partner will need to breathe in lots of short, shallow breaths for a short period of time. Do this with her.

After the head has crowned, your partner can 'breathe' her baby out. This is gentle pushing that comes with breathing into the lower abdomen that will give the head the last little nudge it needs.

When the baby's head crowns, there may be an intense burning sensation for your partner. This is the tissue of the perineum stretching to the max. Some women let out a spectacular scream when this stretching reaches its peak. Then the head will pop out and she's almost there!

Once the head is out, don't be alarmed if your baby doesn't open his or her eyes and say hello. Your baby won't be breathing yet and will probably be looking a pale shade of grey. Tell your partner the head is out and tell her your baby is beautiful. That's all she'll want to hear.

Your caregivers will check to make sure the cord is not wrapped around the baby's neck. It is estimated that this occurs in about 25% of babies. The cord can be easily slipped over the baby's head in the moments prior to the birth. In a small number of cases the cord may be tight, requiring it to be cut to allow the baby to be born. Once the cord is clear, your partner will be asked to give one last gentle push. Your caregivers will guide the baby's shoulder through and then the second shoulder and then the rest of the baby's body will slip out. Like a wet fish, as my mother said.

Get down the business end if you would like to catch your baby, but don't just elbow the midwife or doctor out the way; talk to them about this in advance. Often midwives are happy to facilitate this, especially if you are in a birth centre, but I have often seen obstetricians step aside too and let the father of the child do the 'catching'. If there are no problems with the delivery of your baby, there should be no reason why you can't be the one to do this final step. You'll have to wear gloves but it is pretty cool to be the first person to handle your baby.

Once your baby is out, remember that it is still attached to your partner by the umbilical cord – so don't walk off with the baby in your arms! You should place the baby straight onto your partner's chest.

The moment of birth is a very real end to what can feel like an abstract journey for many dads. Your partner has had this baby growing inside her, changing her chemistry, nudging her from the inside and expanding her belly. It's all been happening to her. But the moment that baby lands Earth-side and you meet your son or daughter, it all becomes very real for you and it can be very emotional.

The fathers I interviewed for this book all said that this moment was incredibly emotional and totally unforgettable. I've seen many dads – big tough plumbers, powerful barristers and six-foot athletes – burst into tears with the overwhelming joy and relief that comes with the moment their baby is born and they realise that their partner is safe and it's all over. I get teary just writing about it.

'The day that my first baby was born was undoubtedly the best day of my life,' says John Keogh who has delivered over 7000 babies in his 25 year career. 'When I held my daughter in my arms for that first moment, it was completely overwhelming. I wanted to go to every room in the hospital and show off my baby girl, this miracle who was now in my arms! I would have laid down my life for her there and then without a second thought. I was as high as a kite with joy. I had delivered many babies before my children were born but when it was my wife in labour, it was a very different experience. I'm still in awe of that miraculous moment of birth when I deliver a baby but I'll never forget the day my own babies were born.'

Brace yourself for the emotional impact of becoming a father, but don't worry if you don't immediately feel over the moon. For some, the buzz just comes later. Those feelings can also be postponed if the moment of birth isn't a perfectly smooth one.

The first few moments of a baby's life are truly miraculous. In the seconds after the baby is born, the fluid that has been in the lungs is suddenly absorbed into the baby's bloodstream to free up the lungs for air. The baby takes a first breath and bingo! He or she has made the amazing transition from an internal, liquid environment to an external one where air is the giver of life.

After the birth, the health of your baby may seem to take over from your partner's health and you may feel ignored by the staff while they check that all is well with your child. If they have to take the baby off to the crib on the other side of the room for some oxygen, stay with your partner. Your baby is in good hands and will be returned to you once all is well.

The main things to remember about the pushing stage and the moment of birth are:

- *Most first babies need to be pushed out with great effort*
- *You have about two hours to produce this baby without intervention, in keeping with hospital protocol, so don't waste time trying to 'breathe' a first baby out*
- *Help your partner into a comfortable position, preferably on all fours or on her side*
- *Whisper encouragement to her between contractions so that you can override any negative medico-speak in the room*
- *Help her get her mojo with a pushing technique that locks off the air in her throat for maximum power*
- *Kiss your partner and tell her you love her*
- *Encourage your partner to relax her pelvic floor and her jaw*
- *When the head crowns, breath with her in little shallow breaths*
- *Get down the business end if you want to catch your baby*
- *Brace yourself for the emotional impact of becoming a father*
- *Once your baby is born, stay close to your partner*

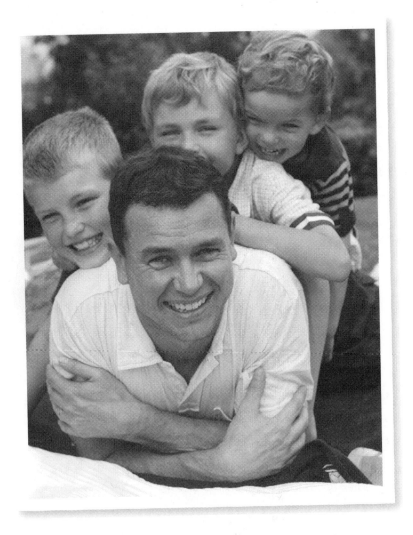

MARK FERGUSON'S STORY

Those last few moments before Jack was born were some of the rawest moments of my life. Memorable, staggering and emotional.

Mark Ferguson is a country boy from Tamworth who started out in regional television over 25 years ago. As a news and current affairs reporter, he's reported everything, from cattle prices to cricket, country music to armed conflicts, eventually presenting the national news bulletin for Nine and Seven. Mark met his English-born wife Jayne on a trip to the Whitsundays to follow a story. Then a five-year stint as a foreign correspondent in London with his new wife saw Mark covering major stories such as the Rwanda massacres, the Palestinian Intifada, the ongoing troubles in Northern Ireland and the death of Diana, Princess of Wales. Mark is the national ambassador for Good Beginnings, a charitable organisation that helps young families adjust to parenthood – an adjustment that Mark refers to as the steepest learning curve of his life.

The birth of my first son Jack was the most amazing day of my life. I was a London correspondent at the time, covering the Ashes. We were told by lots of people, including a London cabbie, that we were having a girl. We were also told by the midwives that our baby would probably be coming early so with three weeks until our due date, my wife Jayne needed to keep off her feet and get as much rest as possible. I took time off work and missed one of the cricket tests so that I would be around for what we were assured would be an early arrival. Jack was born eleven days after his due date. That was 32 days of waiting for him to hatch. Over a month of waiting that became very wearing.

When Jayne went into labour, at last, I was uncertain and nervous about what was to come. We went into Chelsea Westminster Hospital in London in the early stages of labour. After about six hours it was game on and we were moved to the birthing unit.

We had arrived at the hospital at midday and Jack was born at 4am the following day. At one point, I was starving so I went across the road to get some chicken and chips. I came back to the birthing unit and was eating my take-away when Jayne's waters broke. I wasn't very popular for that chicken and chips moment.

The system in the UK is very different from the set up in Australia. It's very midwife-driven in the UK. The midwives were absolutely fantastic when we had Jack. They were caring and nurturing whilst maintaining control. Jayne's best mate from school was with us but she stepped out right at the end and left us to it. I was holding Jayne's hand, helping her to remember the breathing techniques that we had learned in the classes and staying close.

What amazed me most was Jayne's strength through it all. The tougher the labour got, the tougher she got. She was amazing, incredible. Seeing her in pain and not being able to save her from that was hard for me. I was worried that Jayne didn't have a high tolerance for pain but I was stunned by her determination, tolerance and resilience in labour.

Pushing out a nine and a half pound baby was hard work for my wife. I found it difficult to watch Jayne go through that, to push through the pain. Part of a husband's job is to be the protector but I just had to hold her, support and comfort her. Those last few moments before Jack was born were some of the rawest moments of my life. Memorable, staggering and emotional.

I'll never forget that moment. Throughout the pregnancy I had watched Jayne's belly grow and had been involved in preparing for the birth but the reality of it didn't actually hit me until the moment he was born. The emotion, the shock and the surprise were just incredible! For a start, we were expecting a girl and here I had a son staring back at me. He was perfect.

Nothing in my professional life could really prepare me for the role I had to play when I supported Jayne through the birth. I've been in some tense situations, reported from war zones and managed the pressure and stress of deadlines, but none of that was as nerve racking as our first birth.

When you go through this with your partner for the first time, you are stepping through a door into a world you really know nothing about and it's a sharp learning curve. It's a powerful bonding experience for you as a couple, to create this little human being together and be there as your child comes into the world.

The first few hours with Jack were the most magical moments of my life. I roamed the corridors of the hospital holding Jack to my chest, promising him the world. It was like a scene from a movie. I was totally besotted with him.

When we were preparing for Jack's arrival, we must have visited every pram shop in London. It was like buying a new car. The first day we took Jack for a walk in our brand new pram, I am not exaggerating when I say that we were worried that the sky would fall in. We were worried about everyday things – the dog a hundred metres away, the car that could mount the pavement, the odd-looking man across the road. The drive home from hospital was nerve racking too. I guess if I could have my time over, I would try to be a bit more laid back, perhaps take a few more deep breaths.

I think your first child paves the way for the second in a lot of ways. The birth was much easier with Ted, even though he was a ten-pounder. We were also a lot more relaxed as parents.

We had Ted in Sydney at North Shore Private after we had come back to Australia and I was working on Good Medicine [*a TV series on Nine*]. Ted was born only about 40 minutes after we made it to hospital.

His birth was completely different – much more intense and so much faster. I was blown away by what Jayne could handle.

When we were preparing for Ted's arrival, we did some 'Second Child' classes at North Shore Private Hospital. They gave us some great advice on how to welcome our second child so that out first child didn't feel left out. When I arrived at the hospital with Jack, Jayne wasn't holding our new baby in her arms. Instead she gave Jack a huge cuddle with lots of special attention. When he was curious and ready to see his baby brother, he went over to the crib and looked at our new family member. The baby had also brought with him a huge Buzz Lightyear, which made the adjustment easier for Jack.

We thought long and hard about having a third child and with two boys, the pressure was on for a girl. Somehow I knew it was going to be another boy. Sure enough, Paddy came screaming into the world four years after Ted was born. At eight and a half pounds, he was our smallest baby.

It was a very special time. Both Jayne and I knew this was our last baby and that really added to the emotion. Jack and Ted were just that little bit older so they were so excited to have a baby brother. To see my three boys together for the first time was unforgettable!

One of the best moments was taking Paddy and Jayne home from hospital. There were now five of us and it really hit me that I had a lot of responsibility. It was up to me to try to provide for and guide these boys as best I could.

I remember putting Paddy in his car seat and the older boys in their boosters. Jayne slowly got into the car. Then I hopped behind the wheel and I turned around and had a good look at my boys. I said to Jayne 'Look at that. Three boys in the back. How the hell did that happen?'

CHAPTER 12

THIRD STAGE OF LABOUR

Once your baby is born, there is still the third stage of labour to get through and that's the delivery of the placenta. The placenta is a big gorgeous organ that has sustained your baby from its beginnings as a tiny collection of cells to its development into this living, breathing human being.

You are still on the job, so don't go anywhere and don't even think about making phone calls for at least a couple of hours.

Be prepared for lots of blood and fluid to come out with the placenta, which is all pretty normal. If your baby has passed meconium (its first poo) in the womb, it may look like a mudslide.

Your partner will probably be given a jab of Syntocinon to the thigh. This is to eject the placenta faster than if you wait for it to separate from the uterus naturally. Some people believe that this drug can mess with a woman's natural oxytocin production, which she needs to get breastfeeding established, so some couples opt to decline the injection.

If you and your partner really do not want the injection, you should make this known in writing before the birth and you should remind your partner's midwife sometime during labour.

The placenta usually comes out with just one or two pushes from your partner. It shouldn't require much traction on the cord and it usually just plops out into a kidney dish. From your partner's perspective it should feel soft, warm and squishy coming through the birth canal – much more gentle than the baby who came before it. Some women are so taken by their new baby that they barely notice the placenta coming through the birth canal.

You can cut the cord if you wish. Some medical practitioners see value in allowing the cord to stop pulsating before it is cut. The cord provides another lifeline to the baby while breathing is established so some consider that to cut it immediately cuts off a crucial lifeline. Research[1] has shown that delaying cord cutting by just a few minutes gives your baby additional iron-rich cord blood. It can take anywhere from a few minutes to half an hour for the cord to stop pulsating. If the decision is to wait to cut the cord, make sure you check a part of the cord that is slack. If the cord is pulled tight, it will appear to have no pulse already.

There may be some repair to be done if your partner has suffered a tear or was given an episiotomy (surgical cut to the perineum). Over 44% of women birthing for the first time have a tear to the perineum and a further 22% are given a surgical cut[2]. This depends on where a woman gives birth, with private hospitals in most states of Australia having a much higher rate of episiotomy than public hospitals. Very few episiotomies are performed in homebirths.

These statistics add up to a whopping 66% of women birthing for the first time who require some kind of repair work after their baby is delivered.

For many women, tearing is the next biggest fear after the pain of childbirth. It sounds hideous! Imagine your scrotum tearing under pressure. But you can tell your partner from me that there is so much action going on down there with the tissue so stretched out and lacking in blood flow that she won't feel anything more than a powerful burning sensation. It's also important to note that by the time a woman is ready to give birth, the hormone named relaxin has been working its magic for months, loosening her ligaments and especially the birth canal to make it nice and stretchy.

I tore for all three of my births – one being a third degree tear – and

I didn't really feel any of them. I was lucky to avoid going to theatre for that third degree tear. For each of my births, I was surprised when I was told that I would need some stitches, especially my last birth. I hadn't felt anything but a burning sensation.

Repair work can take anywhere from half an hour to 90 minutes or more. Your partner will be given a local anaesthetic, which will really sting and then after that, your job is to distract her with her beautiful baby. Tell her what a legend she is. Kiss her. Again.

You may have heard tacky jokes that this is the time you should ask the doctor to add an 'extra stitch', just to tighten things up so that you'll have greater pleasure with your wife in years to come. I can't think of anything that could make you more unpopular with your partner than a dumb-arse joke like that.

I supported a woman who was a history teacher and when her stitches were being done, she said to her husband, 'Does it look like the Battle of the Somme down there?' It's remarkable how quickly a woman's sense of humour returns after her baby is born. But don't even *think* about the 'extra stitch' joke.

For my first birth, the one that involved the third degree tear, I had put absolutely everything I had into birthing our nine-pound boy. When it came to dealing with the lights, stirrups and new doctors to deal with the tear, which took about an hour and a half to stitch up, I had nothing left in me to cope with it and I totally fell apart. I cried and cried. The tear was complicated and two doctors handled it together. At one point, I said to the doctor, 'That really hurts!' He was puzzled. 'What hurts?' he asked. 'Your thumb is pressing on my clitoris!' I shouted. I'm pretty sure I'll never have cause to use that sentence in a room full of people ever again.

As a side story – a few weeks after Hudson was born I was wandering the aisles of our local supermarket, so proud of my new little bundle that I was hoping I would bump into someone I knew so that I could show him off. In the very next aisle, who did I run into? The doctor with the big thumbs!

The other doctor who had worked on that complicated repair had looked after me when I had been admitted to hospital in premature labour at about 34 weeks, which was stalled for another month so I could give birth at full term. He had to do a vaginal exam and while he's right in the middle of it, shining a yellow Dolphin torch right up there, with Bruce by my side finding it a bit weird but coping, the doctor says to me, 'Did you go to Turramurra Public School?' I nearly died! I did go to Turramurra Public School but I didn't remember this guy from the playground! Bruce was slightly horrified too and said, 'Why? Can you tell by her cervix?'

Back to the repair: Bruce did a great job of distracting me, holding our baby nice and close for me to touch his face. We decided on a name for our son and tried to talk about anything but the commotion going on 'down there'.

Your partner may begin to shake, which is caused by the natural, immediate hormonal let-down after the birth. The midwife may offer some warm blankets to help, but shaking is perfectly normal. You may be shaking too!

Some people like to keep the placenta and bury it under a tree that is planted in the name of the baby. I had a friend who was renting so she planted her baby's placenta at the bottom of a plant pot and grew a citrus tree in the pot. The only problem was that when she watered it, the pot plant 'bled'! Some people like to make a print on paper of the placenta (with the blood that is naturally on the placenta or with paint) to keep some kind of visual record of it.

Some people think this is complete lunacy. It's just a great big, dead organ, no longer required and destined for the hospital incinerator. You decide.

If you would like to keep the placenta, make sure this is written in your notes and remind your caregivers so that they can freeze it for you to take home in a few days' time.

Many cultures see a great significance in this life-giving organ. In some cultures it is even eaten.

For our homebirths, we put the placenta in the freezer with the prawn heads and it went out with the next load of garbage. At the time we had a big dog and knew it would be his next meal if we buried it in the garden.

Some people practise what is referred to as a Lotus Birth. This is where the cord is not cut but is allowed to wither naturally. This takes seven to ten days if it is allowed to remain dry. However, it means the mother has to carry the placenta around with the baby, usually in a little cloth bag, until the cord has withered. In the heat of summer, this means salting the organ. In Iceland, where I doubt they would need to salt the organ, Lotus Birth is common practice.

If you have asked to delay the cutting of the cord and you're not practising Lotus Birth, this is the time when your caregivers will clamp the cord in two places and hand you a pair of surgical scissors for you to make the cut.

The main things to remember during the third stage of labour are:

- *Don't go anywhere or make phone calls: you're still on the job*
- *Cut the cord if that floats your boat*
- *If your partner needs stitches, distract her from the process with your beautiful baby*
- *Ask the hospital to freeze the placenta if you would like to take it home with you*

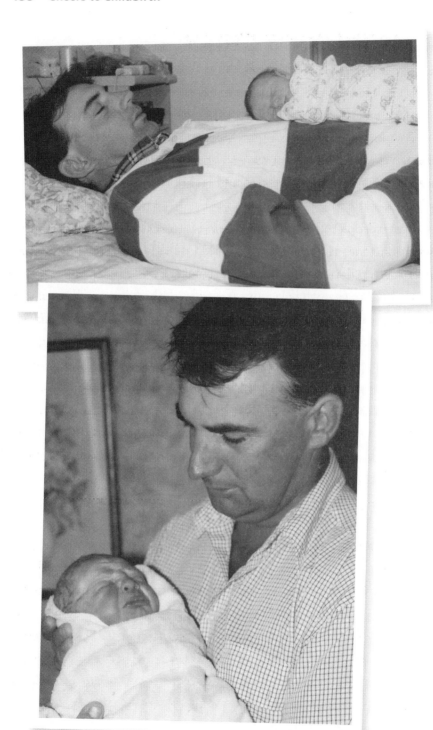

TIM VINCENT'S STORY

Seeing cows calve gave me no help whatsoever in knowing what to expect when my babies were born!

Tim Vincent is a second-generation cattle farmer from the Tamworth region of northern New South Wales. The second of four children, he grew up on the family property and went to school in Tamworth, left at 16 to go to agricultural college and always planned to be a career farmer. He worked on properties in Queensland and then travelled overseas, driving from Texas to Canada, working on cattle properties along the way. Back in Australia, Tim met his wife Margaret, an embryologist working with a stud cattle embryo transfer company. They now run an 800-hectare property with about 500 head of cattle, selling 60 to 70 bulls each year through their stud, Booragul Angus, as well as running a grain-growing enterprise and a feedlot business. Together they have two children who were born almost as simply as a cow births her calf...

When my wife and I got married we were in our late twenties and decided after a year of marriage that it was time to start our family. How easy... Margaret fell pregnant in the first month of trying. We had only just bought our property and at that time it was very old and in need of a lot of work. However, we had to make do at least for a little while until we could afford to renovate, so we did the basics, like a touch of paint here and there. It's amazing what you can achieve in a short time when a baby is on the way. Looking back, Margaret always says the only time anything ever got done was when she was pregnant.

Although Tamworth is a fairly large country town, it really has an incredible shortage of good doctors and that includes obstetricians. We have one private hospital in town and only one doctor who is able to deliver babies there. In saying that, the doctor was great, the hospital was lovely and the staff brilliant, so we were glad we had made sure that we were well covered by health insurance.

We did the usual prenatal classes, which I found really interesting. It was fun to meet some of the other couples who were also mainly from farming backgrounds, swapping stories of how they were trying desperately to get their old farm houses up to scratch in time for the arrival of that special addition to the family.

I didn't read any books, but my wife bought every book in Australia on childbirth. I think she still buys them and we finished having kids a while ago! I figured that I've watched cows calve all my life, so surely reading a book wasn't going to tell me anything I didn't already know about the birth process.

I'm 40 so I've been doing this for 25 years and can spot which two heifers will give birth that day out of a mob of 50. I generally have the heifers all shut in the front paddock so I can keep an eye on them and I get used to spotting the ones who will calve that day. The mob might be gathered all on one side of the paddock with one heifer fidgeting by herself, she may be not be eating or will go to have a drink and then change her mind. They appear to be uncomfortable and restless. Generally they manage things incredibly well and only occasionally do I have to intervene and help nature along a little by pulling the calf out myself. I'm amazed at how quickly and simply a cow can calve. I might take the kids down to the bus and notice a cow fidgeting and by the time I get back, she's had the calf.

However, seeing cows calve gave me no help whatsoever in knowing what to expect when my babies were born!

Margaret had gestational diabetes so she was induced on her due date because this condition produces unusually large babies. She isn't a big woman but her belly certainly had some size to it by her due date.

It was a Tuesday morning and we had to be at the hospital by 8am, which meant leaving home early and driving fairly fast. (When Margaret was told that her blood pressure was a little high on our arrival at the hospital, she blamed it on my driving.) The doctor arrived shortly after we did and broke Margaret's waters. It was full on straight away and three hours later, Amy was born. I would say short and sweet, although Margaret would probably say hard and fast. We had a couple of really good midwives who looked after us, one was the 'Nazi' type and the other was the 'gently does it' kind. As a team they worked well.

In the prenatal classes they had mentioned the spa bath, massage machines, music, massage oil, but not much of that was used. Put simply, there just wasn't any time to spa bath. The labour just seemed to roll on smoothly and quickly; however, Margaret did find that listening to her favourite CD helped her to relax and focus. I just did as Margaret asked. I handed her juice, then the vomit bowl, then the gas, juice, vomit bowl, gas and so it went. I didn't really do anything, to be honest. My major role was just to be there for support. You can't really appreciate the huge amount of pain your wife is going through. They say you haven't experienced pain until you've experienced childbirth.

When Amy was born I felt great relief that everything was all right and that Margaret and the baby were both alive and well. You hear some terrible stories, so I was just so glad that it had all worked out well.

Amy was born in July when it was freezing cold. It even came close to snowing, so Margaret stayed in hospital where it was warm and comfortable for a good five or six days. I travelled back and forth between home and the hospital, which are about 80 kilometres apart. I'd do what I had to do around the place at home and then try to be back at the hospital by mid-morning. The tiredness is something I wasn't prepared for. I expected it when the baby came home but didn't realise how tiring it would be just keeping things going at home, as well as travelling everyday to visit Mum and bub.

Amy was born with a dislocated hip, which is a genetic problem in my family, but it wasn't picked up until she was about five months old. She had been in hospital for an unrelated illness and while she was there they discovered her hip problem, so less than a week before her first Christmas we were rushed to Sydney for Amy to have surgery followed by a full body plaster for three months. This was a really trying time. It was mid summer and stinking hot – 40 degrees or more in Tamworth. When she came out of theatre on a trolley with her legs splayed out in a full body cast, it was the toughest thing, not being able to cuddle our baby close and not knowing if it would even work. We couldn't sit her in a high chair, give her a bath or use a stroller. It was the worst thing at the time but it seems minor when I look back on it now. Two years ago she swam in the state swimming titles and we've all forgotten that her dislocated hip had ever happened.

We had wanted our children to be two years apart and Margaret fell pregnant again, this time in the second month of trying, so it seemed we had that part all worked out. However, this time she didn't feel too well and collapsed at the doctor's with a ruptured ectopic pregnancy. I was there within an hour and there were a couple of very ordinary days to follow after that. This certainly slowed down our plans for a second baby. One of Margaret's fallopian tubes was removed after the ectopic pregnancy and the other was blocked from adhesions, so to have another baby we had to use IVF. Margaret's background in IVF was the best thing going for us. Our son Hayden was a fresh embryo implanted and it took straight away. The rest is history. Just one round of IVF.

During the pregnancy, Margaret grew very, very large, as she had with Amy. We went in for a check-up two weeks before Margaret was due; the doctor checked her out and said she was already four centimetres dilated! We walked across the road to the hospital, they broke her waters and Hayden was born only about an hour later. Hardly enough time for me to fill out my meal menu! That is a running joke with Margaret and me, as whilst she was trying to get a midwife to help push the baby out I was busy trying to decide if I wanted a prawn cocktail or soup for tea.

Margaret doesn't muck around when she has babies and I am very glad she has never gone into labour on our property. We were blessed to be in town both times, right when Margaret was ready for labour and lucky to have had both of our babies at a civilised hour, with no middle of the night run to hospital.

I felt a fair bit of relief again, to know that all was well. Hayden was about seven and half pounds and had a really squashed face that required some physio work for a few weeks. We lived on tenterhooks with Hayden for a few years as he suffered chronic bronchiolitis, then asthma and a diagnosis of sleep apnoea, so he had to be on monitors for a fair while. Thankfully, as he has grown older and stronger he appears to have grown out of most of his problems and is now a bullet-proof kid. We blame the very dusty old home for a lot of his breathing difficulties, but that has all changed now and we have just finished renovating the entire house. Perhaps if Hayden had been healthier when he was little, we might have considered having more children.

What do they say? Kids are the best contraceptive? Maybe, but I wouldn't swap mine for the world.

CHAPTER 13

AFTER THE BIRTH: THE FIRST FEW HOURS

The moments and hours after the birth of your baby are very important. You are still the protector of the birthplace, so defend it! This is why it's best not to broadcast to family and friends that you are even in labour. If you do, by the time your partner gives birth, especially if it is a long labour, the grandparents of your baby may be tapping their toes in the waiting room and you may feel pressured to let them in to see your baby.

I have attended births where all four grandparents were in the waiting room of the birthing unit at three in the morning, waiting to see their grandchild. I wanted to tell them to go home and knit something. They weren't doing any good there, other than making the couple feel pressure to produce the baby before Grandpa had a stroke from the stress of it all.

The best-case scenario is if you have your baby in the middle of the night, then you don't need to tell anyone until the morning. This will give you a few hours to bond with your baby and get breastfeeding established. Remember – you have a new family now. However, best-case doesn't always happen and even if your baby is born at midday, the rest of the family (even if you are from a huge extended family) can wait.

Some birth professionals believe that the first 24 hours of your baby's life is so critical that this time should not be shared with anyone outside your new family unit. This might sound harsh, but you will never get back that time with your baby. Your in-laws can pass the baby around like a football *after* you have bonded with your baby, established a good feeding routine and given your partner a chance to clean herself up and have some rest.

I think it is better to save visitors for when you are at home. That gives you a couple of days to adjust to having this new little family member. Your partner needs space to look after herself and her bub and you need time to establish your role as father in a confident and positive way before you have spectators.

Don't let the midwives rush you into having the newborn procedures done immediately after the birth. These procedures include weighing the baby and measuring body length and head circumference. These things aren't going to change in the next couple of hours so they don't need to be done immediately. Sometimes if there is a shift change, the midwife who helped your partner birth your baby may be keen to finish up her paperwork. That can wait. It's more important that you are all given time to bond as a family.

It's a huge adjustment for this precious, fragile little child to adapt from the protected, quiet, warm, liquid environment of the womb to the noisy, cold, brightly lit world we live in. Keep the lights dim, let your baby hear your gentle voice and cuddle up close.

'In those immediate moments after the birth, another hormone called catecholamine comes into play,' says midwife and academic Hannah Dahlen. 'This hormone makes even the most tired mother become alive and awake and makes her fiercely protective of her newborn. She'll open her eyes and so will her baby, who has the same hormonal surge, and they'll look into each other's eyes and start that critical bonding process.'

Don't let anyone wrap up your baby straight away. Your newborn baby should be given skin-to-skin contact with your partner from the moment of birth. If the midwife does wrap up your baby, just lie your baby on the bed and undo the wrap (remember, this baby belongs to you and your partner) then give your baby to your partner with the blanket on top to keep bubs warm.

Ideally, your baby is put straight onto your partner's bare chest. I've been at births where the doctor or midwife has helped the baby's shoulders out and then the birthing mother has reached down and lifted her baby out herself, putting her baby straight onto her chest.

If you are catching your baby, don't just stand there holding the child! Place your baby on your partner's chest and get up close for a cuddle. Discover your baby's gender and congratulate your partner.

Skin-to-skin contact is a critical aspect of your baby's first hours of life and only in the case of a medical emergency should this be interrupted. Dr Michel Odent has brought together decades of research into this area of neonatal health in his book *The Scientification of Love*. Odent's book[1] indicates that the way a baby is handled in the first hours of life will influence that child's ability to bond, even in adult relationships. Allowing skin-to-skin contact for your partner and baby within the first two hours is critical and should not be passed up lightly.

If your partner can't hold your baby, you are the next best thing. Don't park your baby in the crib. Take off your shirt and cuddle your newborn to your chest, with a blanket around you both. Newborns don't have very good temperature control in their little bodies so you will need to keep your bub warm, especially in a cold hospital environment. Your baby is already familiar with your voice, so talk gently, stroke their skin, kiss their little head. Tell them you love them. Tell them all about the adventures you have planned for the next twenty years or so.

Make sure that you stay by your partner's side and let her enjoy her baby too.

A newborn's sense of smell is well developed and they will use that sense to find the mother's breast for their first feed.

Give your partner something to eat if she wants it. Her senses are heightened so the first thing she eats after giving birth often tastes like the best meal in the world. Your senses are heightened too as you'll also be in cave man protector mode and many men report that the first thing they eat after their baby is born tastes fantastic.

Give your partner space and time to establish breastfeeding. This is a whole new challenge and she'll need your support to help get breastfeeding happening. Your baby's first feed should ideally happen within an hour or so of the birth.

Your partner needs to make one of her nipples available to your baby, holding your baby close to its new food source so that the sense of smell will help guide the way while maintaining skin-to-skin contact. A little massage of the nipple and a gentle squeeze from behind the nipple will produce some colostrum, the watery golden liquid that your partner will produce for the first few days before her milk comes in.

Once your baby starts to crane for the breast and nuzzle your partner's chest, it's time to pop your partner's entire nipple inside the baby's mouth. This is easier said than done. It usually takes several attempts to get this right. Some babies get the gist straight away, others take some time. If you need help, ask a midwife to assist but this help should be gentle and the midwife should ask before she touches your partner's breasts. Once the baby has attached to the nipple well, with a good strong sucking mechanism in place, you're in business.

Don't let your partner feed for too long on the same breast. She will damage her nipples if she feeds for more than about 15 minutes on each side. She will need to use her little finger to break the suction of the baby's mouth before switching sides. If she pulls the baby off without breaking this strong suction, it will really hurt! See Chapter 16 for further details on breastfeeding and how you can support your partner in this challenging part of early motherhood.

Breastfeeding produces oxytocin, which contracts the uterus and for some women, especially those birthing for the second or third time, this produces after birth pains, which are very painful. These pains usually only occur while breastfeeding and only for the first couple of days. After my second and third babies were born, the after birth pains were spectacular. They rivalled the actual labour pains! My friend Melinda discovered the best treatment for after birth pains when she gave birth to her third child – a suppository of strong analgesic immediately after the birth. 'I'm not putting up with after birth pains after everything I have been through!' said Melinda. 'I *asked* for the suppository after I had my fourth child.'

If your partner has had stitches, it is really important that she doesn't get dehydrated or constipated for the next few days. Make sure she is drinking plenty of water – more than usual and offer her a fibre drink like Metamucil within a couple of hours of the birth.

You'll have to wait on your partner hand and foot if she has had an epidural as this can take several hours to wear off. There was a case in the US where a woman tried to get out of bed before the epidural had worn off completely and fell over and broke her leg! I can't imagine how hard it would be to look after a newborn with a leg in plaster.

Your baby is usually born covered in a magic white goo called vernix. Make sure that you leave the vernix on your baby's skin. Don't strip off this beautiful natural moisturiser with soap products that are completely unnecessary at this stage of your baby's life. Your baby has lived in a liquid environment all this time and the vernix will sink in over the next couple of hours and nourish it in a way that no man-made product ever could. If there is a build up of vernix in some of the deeper creases such as under the arms and at the groin, wipe this away if it hasn't naturally been absorbed into the skin within a couple of hours.

In some hospitals, midwives are keen to bath your baby so that they know they have shown you how to do this properly. Your baby does not need to be bathed every day and should not be bathed at all until the little umbilical stump has dried up and dropped off. This takes seven to ten days to come away naturally but if you keep wetting the stump by bathing your baby, it will take three or four weeks to come off. The stump smells like rotting flesh so it's not something you'll want to hang on to for a month if you can avoid it.

It is usual procedure in Australian hospitals for newborns to be given an injection of vitamin K to prevent a rare condition called Haemorrhagic Disease of the Newborn (HDN). If you do not want this injection, make sure the midwife is aware of this. You can opt for an oral version of the vitamin but it is trickier to administer to such a young baby, which is why the injection is the norm.

After giving birth, your partner will bleed. At first it will be heavy bleeding and then it will be lighter and about six weeks after the birth it should be all finished. Help your partner to have a warm shower in the first few hours after the birth. If she uses incontinence briefs (as recommended in your hospital packing list in Chapter 8) rather than maternity pads in her underwear, it will save you taking home washing to do. These briefs are well padded and comfortable to wear if your partner has had stitches. One pack of incontinence pants will see your partner through the heaviest bleeding and then she can switch to maternity pads once she's at home.

Once your baby is born, everyone pays attention to the baby, the baby, the baby. So make sure that you are paying special attention to your partner. Ask her how she's feeling. Remember that adrenalin blocks the oxytocin that she needs to breastfeed successfully so make sure she is happy, comfortable and relaxed. Keep up your role as protector of this family.

People will bring mountains of stuff for your baby, especially when you have your first child. So make sure you give something special to your partner that isn't a size 0000 designed for your baby.

I have three words for you boys: DAY SPA VOUCHER. Every woman loves a pampering after giving birth. Actually, those three words will get you out of trouble at any time in your life! You could also give her a nice pair of pyjamas – she'll be spending a fair bit of time in them over the next few weeks. This is not the time for sexy lingerie. That will only get you into trouble.

You may feel somewhat neglected during this time as your partner (and everyone else) pays so much attention to your baby. Get over it. Her attention will be divided between you and your children forevermore. You'll just have to get used to the new status quo. However, you have a shared experience and this wonderful new baby that can bring you closer together as a couple. Her undivided attention to your baby is not permanent. There is light at the end of the tunnel and she'll be able to give you the love and attention you crave when she's not hormonally driven to fend for and feed this tiny, dependent newborn.

If there's only one thing you remember from this chapter, let this be it: bonding is critical and your baby needs skin-to-skin contact immediately after the birth. This should not be interrupted unless there is a medical emergency. The other things worth remembering, but not as critical to your baby's health, are:

- *You are still the protector of the birthplace*
- *Don't call family or friends for at least a few hours*
- *Give your partner the space and support to start breastfeeding*
- *Leave the natural vernix to sink into your baby's skin*
- *Don't feel rushed into newborn procedures*
- *Pay special attention to your partner, not just the baby*

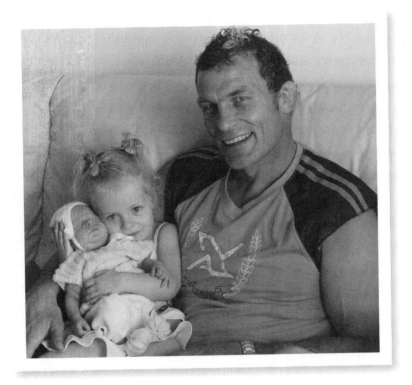

JUD ARTHUR'S STORY

It was one of the best experiences of my life seeing that wee head crowning and coming out. It was just amazing.

Jud Arthur has an interesting combination of talents. He played professional rugby in Italy and in his homeland of New Zealand, played state level basketball and represented New Zealand in show jumping. Whilst recuperating from the knee injury that ended his sporting career, Jud rekindled his passion for singing and in particular, opera. After some amateur musical society roles and without any formal training, Jud won the lead role of Angelotti in a New Zealand Opera production of Tosca. He is now one of Australia's leading bass-baritones, working for Opera Australia and other professional opera companies here and across the Tasman, performing in productions such as Madame Butterfly, Aida, La Boheme, The Mikado, Midsummer Night's Dream, Les Miserables and Carmen. Jud has worked as a fashion model and a butcher and has competed in body building competitions. He is also a qualified horse farrier, shoeing horses between opera performances. Together with his wife Nicky, an author and a yoga and meditation instructor, Jud has two young daughters, Lucia and Millijana. According to Jud, his girls have brought out his softer side.

Nicky and I met at the rugby. We were married about ten months after we first met and competed in pairs competitions in body building. I was ready to settle down when I met Nicky. Three years later, we had Lucia.

When Lucia was born I was performing in Wellington. Nicky and I had planned for a natural birth and had done a lot of preparation together with meditation, relaxation and visualisations. Nicky had some tapes that we worked through. She programmed her body to handle the pain and I was able to use those techniques to talk her through and keep her calm with deep breathing exercises and visualisations. We practised this during the pregnancy.

It's hard for a guy to really feel like he's doing much that's useful during the labour. I think that just being there is supportive. I would have done anything to make sure I didn't miss the birth.

Nicky was so calm and brave. She was fantastic. I had confidence in her that she could handle it. I knew she'd be able to do it. She's a very positive person with a lot of determination.

It was one of the best experiences of my life seeing that wee head crowning and coming out. It was just amazing. It was exhilarating and I couldn't wipe the smile off my face! I was on cloud nine and was going around saying, 'I've just had a baby! A beautiful baby girl!'

Lucia was the most beautiful thing I'd ever seen. We didn't know whether we were having a boy or a girl and it was a wonderful surprise, although I didn't even think to look for her gender in the moments after she was born. This beautiful baby had arrived and I was just so taken with that. It wasn't until the midwife said, 'You have a beautiful baby girl,' that I thought, 'Oh, wow!'

Lucia's birth was only about seven hours long. It was so straightforward and Nicky did such a great job. After the birth I went across the road to the deli and bought her salmon sandwiches, soft cheeses and some of the other things that she hadn't been allowed to eat while she was pregnant. She wolfed it down!

We took life with a newborn in our stride, I think. Nicky's mum came up for the first week to help out and give Nic some emotional support. Nic is a very capable woman. She thinks that being a mother doesn't come naturally to her, but I think she's a great mother. Only a few weeks later, we moved to Australia.

Three years after Lucia was born we had Millijana. Hers was a different story. We had just bought our house in Sydney and I had signed on to perform a season of The Magic Flute for Opera Australia in Melbourne. We decided to induce the labour so that we could have Millijana two weeks before her due date and then pack up and move down to Melbourne in time for the season to start.

I was flying backwards and forwards, performing in Melbourne and coming back to Sydney to look after my horse-shoeing clients in the weeks before the birth. Moving house on top of having a baby was pretty stressful. Nicky handled things well, but this was a challenging time.

Nicky's body wasn't ready for the labour and Millijana wasn't ready to be born either. The baby was distressed but Nic wasn't dilating. About four hours after the induction, the doctor said we should have a Caesarean. We felt like he knew what he was doing.

I had a good look at what was going on during the surgery. I grew up on a farm and I've worked in the chain as a butcher, so blood and guts don't bother me, but this was my wife and baby so it was quite overwhelming. It was almost like an out of body experience.

God help us if men had to go through childbirth.

Nic recovered fantastically from the Caesarean. A lot of women struggle but Nic is very fit. She's an unstoppable force! Two weeks later she was back into it and we made the move to Melbourne a couple of weeks after that.

That is one thing I would do differently. We should have told the opera company that I would be late and then let Nicky give birth in her own time.

Having children has added a lot of depth and meaning to my life. I'm responsible for these children for life and that's a big deal. It has changed my outlook. Being a father has also helped me characterise fathers a lot better in my opera roles!

I went into fatherhood thinking I would have a hard line approach to discipline: that I would be able to lay down the law and that the kids would obey. It doesn't work like that. You have to be good at listening to your kids. They love it when you listen to them, even from a very young age. I didn't do that early on and it used to frustrate the hell out of Lucia. I could have been a bit softer.

I didn't have a father, it was just me and my mum growing up. I was a spoilt little bugger and I had to get over that, but I didn't want my kids to be spoilt like I was. Without a father figure I didn't have a role model for how a father should behave. I just had to think on my feet and learn as I went. I just had to be me: soft but firm. They're both very loving wee girls and we're very blessed.

CHAPTER 14

CAESAREANS

There is more than a 30% chance that your partner will have a Caesarean. About half of these are couples who have no intention of birthing their baby in an operating theatre. This is an incredibly high national average when the World Health Organisation states that no region in the world justifies a Caesarean rate higher than 10-15%. The Caesarean rate in Finland is just over 15% – the lowest of all developed countries. Some Australian hospitals have rates over 60%!

A Caesarean brings its own risks with it. It is major abdominal surgery and poses documented medical risks to your partner and your baby. However, Caesareans also save lives. The trick is choosing caregivers who will make this decision with great caution, while you have enough knowledge to be sure that you won't allow yourselves to be pushed into an unnecessary procedure.

Some couples choose to have an elective Caesarean for a number of reasons, usually none of which concern the baby's health. Some people like the predictability of knowing precisely when the baby will be born so they can plan their lives around it. Many women fear vaginal birth so much that a surgical alternative is a less frightening option.

For some women who have laboured naturally and then have to face an unscheduled Caesarean, the operation represents the height of failure. They have 'failed' to birth their baby naturally. This is a major issue for some women, with support groups to help them recover from the trauma of a surgical delivery.

'I had some hypnosis and various natural preparations for birth,' says my friend Sharon. 'I'm a natural therapist so I thought birth was an entirely natural event. When we were faced with a Caesarean after three days of labour and a baby in distress, I was *gutted*. If I see a birth on TV, I still cry and six years later my husband thinks we should have another baby so that a vaginal birth could heal these wounds. Perhaps then I'll be complete.'

Some men also feel let down that the experience they had hoped to share with their partner is replaced by a trip to theatre.

In this situation, you need to assure your partner that she is still giving birth, that she's an amazing woman to have nurtured this baby inside her body and that she will be a fantastic mother. Remind her that this will save the baby's life and end this protracted labour so that you can welcome your baby into the world. Your partner is still giving birth and will still be a mother at the end of the day. Sing Happy Birthday to the baby if you have to.

On the other hand, some women have no problem at all with having a Caesarean. My friend Nic had an easy natural birth for her first child followed by an unscheduled Caesarean for her second. 'I'd happily have a Caesarean again. It was great! I was very fit at the time and recovered quickly.'

Your partner will have a spinal anaesthetic or epidural in preparation for the operation. If she hasn't already had an anaesthetic and the procedure is extremely urgent, she'll be given a general anaesthetic and in some hospitals, you won't be permitted in the room for the surgery.

My bookkeeper Darren was not allowed in theatre for the Caesarean births of each of his two sons. His wife had a general anaesthetic so Darren waited outside until their little bundle was handed to him. Darren says the moment where he met his new child was 'magic' and that being excluded from theatre didn't have any effect on bonding with his boys.

Obstetrician Dr John Keogh says, 'I really want the father to be present in theatre for a Caesarean birth, even when his partner has had to have a general anaesthetic. It is after all, still the birth of his baby and a very special occasion. He is there to support his partner but that's not the only reason. He's about to be a new dad!'

Usually, once the decision has been made to perform the operation, you will be transferred to theatre promptly. You won't have to scrub up but you will have to put on theatre clothes that look like pyjamas.

If your partner ends up on the operating table to have her baby, there is much to be learned from this woman's experience:

'I had an emergency Caesarean – the kind where there is no time for an epidural so the procedure had to be with a general anaesthetic. It was all a big rush and the theatre nurse told my bewildered husband to go to the room next door, put on a theatre gown and hurry back. I'd been labouring for days and we were both completely strung out and exhausted. As the medical staff were quickly preparing me for the procedure, my husband returned, backing in through the theatre doors so as not to touch them with his gloved hands. The last thing I remember as I went under the powerful sedative of a general anaesthetic was the sight of my husband's hairy arse poking out the back of his theatre gown. He had taken off all his clothes before putting on the gown!'

The moral to this story is: keep your duds on.

It only takes about ten minutes from the time the surgery starts to the time the baby is born. Have your camera ready because it all happens very quickly.

It is full on surgery so if this bothers you, don't look at the gory end. There will be a drape up between your partner and the action so you don't have to see anything you don't want to. If, however, this fascinates you, watch your baby being born, but remember you are there to support your partner so hold her hand and tell her what's happening in a gentle way, not in a 'Phwooor! Look at that!' kind of way.

My friend Barry 'fesses up, as only Barry could, to finding the visuals of a Caesarean more than a little disturbing: 'The huddled experts decided that the baby was getting distressed so Plan C for Caesar was the only choice, with a side dish of epidural. A green tent was hastily erected around most of my wife's body, sort of like a camping trip on the banks of the Birth Canal. Her head was the only visible part, like a tick on a green dog. I stood at her head mopping her brow, wondering why I didn't have a camera with me, when the doctor asked if I'd like to join them inside the hallowed tent. To me, that tent might as well have been surrounded by blue police tape. I declined the offer and stood there gritting my teeth, trying to block out the loud squelching noises before our son was finally born.'

The diathermy or scalpel that the surgeon uses to stop bleeding does produce some smoke and the smell can be a bit off-putting. Don't make a fuss, just be aware that it may bother you. My friend Katrina said after her Caesarean, 'I could swear I smelled smoke and told the doctors that something was burning. I had no idea it was me! Crikey.'

It takes a fair bit of pulling and pushing to get the baby out of the pelvic cavity so be prepared for what may seem to be some rough handling of your partner.

Theatre is very cold so your baby will be rubbed up and wrapped in blankets then brought to you for a cuddle. As discussed in the previous chapter, skin-to-skin contact is absolutely crucial to your baby's ability to bond. In the case of a Caesarean, you can ask to have your naked baby placed on your partner's naked chest with blankets covering them to keep them warm. The baby can lie there and gaze into your partner's eyes for the next half hour or so while the surgery is finished.

Once your baby is born, lavish all your attention on your partner and your baby while the surgical team stitches everything back together.

Babies born by Caesarean come out looking beautiful. They haven't been squished by the birth canal (that squished journey actually stimulates the baby's circulation and breathing so it is important) so they usually come out looking pink and perfect.

The birthing mother will go to recovery for observation (remember, she's had major surgery) and this takes about an hour. In most hospitals, you will go with your baby to settle into your room in the maternity ward. If you have a doula, you can request that she go with your partner to recovery. This will help your partner pass the time quickly because she'll be itching to get to her baby. Being in recovery can be a very difficult separation for a mother who is hormonally craving her baby.

Some Australian hospitals have recognised that this separation is very difficult for a woman who has just given birth and allow mother and baby to be together in recovery. Recovery nurses are not trained to care for newborns so a midwife is brought into the recovery room to keep an eye on the baby. Ask your caregivers well in advance if you would like mother and baby to stay together in recovery, to see if they can accommodate this.

If you are not afforded this option, make sure that once your baby has been weighed and measured, NO ONE holds your baby except you until your partner makes it back to the ward. This is why in-laws need to be given their boundaries and preferably not even told that you're in labour, unless you both agree to it beforehand.

I supported a woman who had a Caesarean and by the time she arrived at the maternity ward after her time in recovery, all four grandparents had cuddled her baby before she had had a chance and her baby smelled of her mother-in-law's perfume. She felt that these people had muscled their way in and interfered with her bonding and she didn't bond properly with that child until after her second child was born.

As soon as you make it back to the ward with your baby, take off your shirt, unwrap your baby and lie down with a blanket over you both for the best cuddle of your life and that vital skin-to-skin contact. Don't worry if your baby is crying. That's normal.

Your partner will return from theatre on a good dose of morphine to conquer the pain. Make sure she's comfortable, then tuck the baby in on her chest under her theatre gown and give your baby its first proper skin-to-skin cuddle with Mum, but stay close by as she may be very groggy.

Your partner's recovery from the operation can be much slower than if she had given birth naturally, though this isn't always so if there's been a bad vaginal tear in a normal birth. You will need to wait on her hand and foot for at least a couple of weeks. She won't be able to drive for about six weeks and the heaviest thing she can carry will be your baby. Think carefully before hiring or investing in a capsule style car seat. If your partner has a Caesarean, she won't be able to carry your baby in it.

Your partner's stay in hospital will be longer if she has a Caesarean. It's major abdominal surgery so there is a wound to care for, pain relief drugs to take for a few days or weeks and possibly a general anaesthetic to recover from. On top of this, your partner will be trying to establish breastfeeding and will be adjusting to motherhood and recovering from what she's just been through. She will need your steady, calm, loving support through all of this to help her navigate the first few days of motherhood with a post-operative start. You will probably be totally exhausted, but frankly, there will be little time to catch up on sleep.

Even if you have no intention of having your baby birthed by Caesarean, you should remember these points:

- Assure your partner that she is still giving birth and that she's going to be a fantastic mother
- Put your surgical gear on **over** your clothes
- Don't look down the business end unless you know you can handle it
- Stay close to your partner and let her touch her baby while she's being stitched up
- DO NOT let anyone else hold your baby until your partner returns to the ward and has begun the bonding process

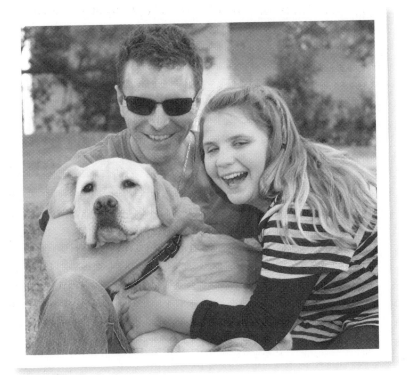

GERRARD GOSENS' STORY

When it came to giving birth, I found that if I kept physical contact with Heather as much as possible, almost wrapped around her, I could feel each contraction and physically support her through it.

Gerrard Gosens has achieved more than most men under forty – yet he's completely blind. He's run numerous marathons and has competed at three Paralympic Games. He's run the 2000km between Brisbane and Cairns five times, reached Mount Everest's Camp Three, co-piloted an ultra light motorglider around Queensland three times and competed in the National Tandem Long Board Surfing Championships. All of this took place while he was Queensland Executive Officer and National Projects Manager of the Australian Paralympic Committee, then Deputy Chief Executive Officer of the Royal Blind Foundation and now Special Projects Manager for Vision Australia. In 2009, in a television world-first, Gerrard faced his greatest challenge ever when he took to the dance floor on Dancing with the Stars, something his two children thought was pretty cool. Now he's competing in the National Latin Dance Championships and planning his next Everest climb.

I met my wife Heather in 1990 when I was running from Brisbane to Cairns through Maryborough. She was walking through the mall at lunchtime and I had been given the honour of firing the canon to mark Heritage Week. Heather came over and talked to me and my dog Joey at the civic reception. I asked her out to dinner and the rest is history. You could say it was a blind date.

When Heather and I had children, my biggest fear was passing on my genetic blindness to my kids. The doctors said there was a 50:50 chance.

When it comes down to it though, blindness is not as challenging as some other disabilities, for example, the experience of having multiple disabilities.

When Heather went into labour with our son Jordon, I was the CEO at the Paralympic Committee and we were at my office. We drove straight to the hospital, but I wish I could have driven her myself.

I found the hospital environment challenging. As a vision impaired person, I rely on my other senses and the smell of hospitals always gets to me. It's also a very cold environment. I couldn't see what was going on around Heather but I could pick up on her voice.

Throughout the pregnancy, I had been very hands-on, touching Heather's belly and feeling our baby growing inside. I loved getting Heather to eat an ice cube and then feeling the baby move away from it.

When it came to the birth, I found that if I kept physical contact with Heather as much as possible, almost wrapped around her, I could feel each contraction and physically support her through it.

I can't give or perceive facial expressions so I can't read Heather's state of mind like someone else can. In Dancing with the Stars, Jess, my dance partner, would say, 'Give me a sultry look,' and I would say, 'I have no idea what that looks like!' Physical contact was what I *could* do to stay in touch with the birth and support Heather throughout the process.

At one point I asked Heather to put her arms around my neck so I could get closer, but when the contraction came, she had me in a tight head lock. That was a mistake! My advice to other men is to make sure your partner has short finger nails. Heather dug her nails into me during contractions and that was certainly painful!

Jordan was a big boy – a ten-pound baby who wasn't going to come out the natural way. Heather is only about five foot tall and weighs 48 kilos. Eventually, she had to have a Caesarean. I found the surgery very distracting. I had to separate myself from the commotion around me – the machinery, the sterility, the smell, the coldness of the beds – and totally support Heather. I found the whole emotional change in environments very sudden. I wish I had been better prepared for the first Caesarean, but it all happened so fast.

The birth of Jordan was a sensational experience. To have been fully sighted would have been even more fantastic. Some men may be fearful of their wife being in pain and may take a step back from it all, but to be there, to share the moment and try to feel that pain with her was awesome. I loved being in the moment with my wife.

I found the first weeks with a newborn pretty easy to adjust to. I wondered if I would be able to care for my baby properly without sight, but those initial fears were quickly overcome. I'm attuned to my sense of hearing so I could quickly work out which cry meant what. I think Heather goes more on the visuals, but I could tell if our kids were ever bunging it on!

Jordan presented a real challenge when he started to crawl. 'Where'd he go?' I would think. I was worried I'd step on him or trip over him. Heather always takes great joy in explaining that I wasn't perfect at changing nappies so I used to give the baby a shower just to make sure he was all clean before putting on a fresh one.

When we had our second child, a little girl called Taylor, all my fears were realised. She inherited my congenital sight problem. She has only four percent sight.

She was a big baby too and so we had a scheduled Caesarean. I was in the operating theatre and they put Taylor in the crib to do her weights and measures. While they fixed Heather up, I was feeling the baby's arms and legs. She grabbed my finger and pulled it closer to her face. I thought immediately, 'Something is wrong here.' The paediatrician confirmed that she did have something wrong with her sight and the news hit me hard. I had to hang on to the sink to stop myself from fainting.

I think vision impairment is harder for a girl. I wondered when she was born about how she was going to put on her make up properly when the time came. Those sorts of delicate girl things worried me, but we have overcome what I call the 'learned fears' and she's a great kid, doing very well.

For the woman, birth is a physical challenge, but as a couple it was an emotional challenge for us. We didn't have our parents nearby so we were in this together as a couple. I wondered what this newcomer would mean to our relationship. The unknowns of childbirth were a challenge too.

When you run a marathon, you swear you'll never, ever put yourself through it again, but within a week you're planning the next one. Childbirth seems to have the same effect on people.

We approached the birth in the same way that I have prepared for climbing Everest or running a marathon or running from Brisbane to Cairns. If you look at the huge challenge ahead in sections, you can handle it. One section at a time.

It took our kids a while to work out that I'm blind. Heather and I used to cheat with little signals so that I could respond to visual things and the kids would wonder how I could 'see' what they were doing. Now that they obviously know that I'm blind, the kids sometimes try to take advantage of it by trying to do something really quietly. But my hearing is very good.

The kids thought their dad being on Dancing with the Stars was great, though Jordan has hit his teens and I thought he might think it was very uncool. One day, for discipline reasons, I had to tell him he couldn't do something he wanted to do and he said right back at me, 'You may be a good dancer, but you suck as a dad!' I thought that was great! He liked my dancing!

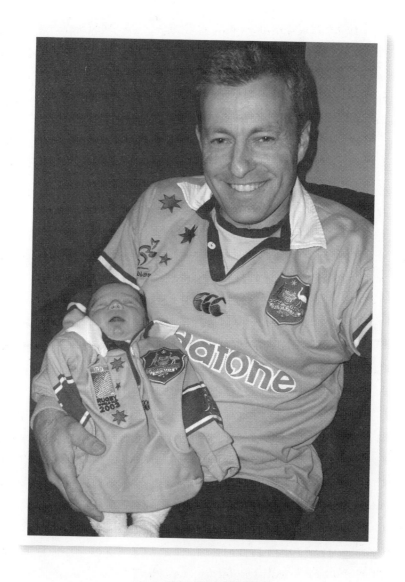

PART THREE

CHAPTER 15
LIFE AFTER BIRTH

Happy Fathers' Day! You are now facing your new role in life, that of a father. With the birth behind you and your baby at home, the lifelong challenge of parenting lies before you. How's that for a daunting prospect?

Many men report an odd sense of concern that they are handed this little child with no instruction manual, no test to pass or interview process to go through in order to prove their aptitude for fatherhood. Together with your partner, you're out on your own and this can feel a little scary.

Once you make it home, you are on a whole new roller coaster ride. Your partner is still an hormonal fruit cake, but she'll be back eventually. She will be fragile in a way you may not have experienced with her before. Many women are also fiercely protective of their baby, almost with a cave woman kind of ferocity. This is normal and healthy. Her attention will return to you eventually but in those first weeks, her baby is her entire world.

Get your act together for the day you bring your partner and baby home from the hospital. Have the house neat and tidy, with a few meals prepared and ready to go so that your partner is not required even to think about cooking meals on top of the demands of your new family member. Your partner will need really good nutrition when she is breastfeeding so relying on too much take-away food is not a good plan.

My brother Michael had a bit of a shindig with his mates just after his first child was born – a little 'wet the baby's head' get-together for the lads. The next day he went to collect his wife and new baby from the hospital and brought them home to a house that smelled of cigar smoke and with a stack of pizza boxes in the kitchen. Needless to say, his wife wasn't too impressed.

A few years later when they gave birth to their second child, Mike had learned his lesson. He had the house neat and tidy, all the laundry was done and he had lunch prepared and in the fridge. When they walked in the door he could open the fridge, pull the plastic wrap off a plate of sandwiches and say, 'Voilà!' That was more like it.

Arrange for extra help around the house if you can. Some help with the washing, cooking, cleaning and grocery shopping will make you and your partner's life easier, giving you more time to look after her and your baby. Accept genuine help when it's offered. Hopefully some meals will land on your doorstep from friends and family too. You can hire a postnatal doula who will help with these chores and can also help with breastfeeding problems and settling techniques for your baby if she's qualified and experienced in these areas.

Most couples find the first six weeks of life with their newborn to be quite a challenge. As my friend Jessica says, 'We all do it tough with newborns, some of us are just better actors than others.' Don't feel that you have to meet others' expectations in dealing with this early parenting challenge and don't feel that you have to socialise either. Your partner needs you more now than ever before. Anyone who tells you that the first weeks of their baby's life were a walk in the park was either residing in another country to said newborn or seriously embellishing the truth. It's exhausting but it's not permanent.

It's not cool to be a klutz with your baby and you are capable of doing everything your partner can with this child, except for breastfeeding, so get involved from day one. If childbirth is not a spectator sport, then neither is parenting. Learn to handle your baby with confidence, something that can only be done with practice.

> **We have a big dog. How do we prepare him for our new family member?**
> A man's best friend comes down a peg on the ladder of love in your household when a baby is born! We had a big, beautiful Weimaraner when we started our family and the vet suggested that we bring home an item of clothing that our baby had worn soon after birth. This gave Murphy the opportunity to familiarise himself with the new scent that would soon dominate our household. He became fiercely protective of our children and was a wonderful guard dog. However, the family hound should never be left alone with your newborn baby. Even if you think your pup is the gentlest breed in the world, you don't want to find out the hard way that he's feeling territorial and wants to silence this attention-getter for good.

People used to ask me how I 'trusted' Bruce to take our baby out on his own. This irritated us both because it suggested that men have no clue as to how to care for their own children and that they're babysitting rather than parenting. Pah! You can be just as capable with and responsible for this child as your partner is.

Manage the visitors who come to your house by putting your partner and baby first. I couldn't believe my eyes the other day when I saw a status update on Facebook from a new father declaring that he and his wife were home from hospital with their new baby and it was open house to all Facebook friends!

One visitor in the morning and one in the afternoon is more than enough and you should try to have a day off in between with no visitors at all. Any more people than this marching through your front door will only exhaust mother and child. Let your visitors know politely when it's time to leave: 'It's been great to see you. Thanks for the visit. Let me see you out so that bub can have the next feed.'

Alternatively you can have an open house a week or ten days after the baby is born. Invite friends and family to come for two hours at the most. Your partner can stay in the bedroom with the baby until everyone has arrived and then she can come out and present your baby to the important people in your life. If you don't want to pass around the baby, have bubs in a baby sling strapped to Mum's chest. Your partner can then go around the room introducing your new family member to each person, one at a time. Once she's had enough, she can vanish to the bedroom to feed your baby and you can thank everyone for coming.

Remember: *This* is your family now. Others' expectations for having a slice of your baby need to be put on hold so that you can look after your partner and your child properly.

Make nappy changes your job. Forever. It's an easy job to do and gives you a chance to have some one-on-one dad time at the change table. It's a great time to have eye contact with your baby. Don't worry about the smell. Babies' poos don't smell until they start eating burgers. Their poos start out being black (like Vegemite) for a few days and then they go a mustard yellow colour (like peanut butter).

Once the cord stump had fallen off, I bathed our babies with me in the bath, holding them in my arms. Then Bruce would take the baby from me to do the drying and dressing. This gave me the opportunity to have a peaceful soak in the bath and Bruce the chance to have some more one-on-one time with our bub. He taught all three of our babies to roll over during these post-bath dad sessions.

Keep an eye out for the 'baby blues'. On about day three after the birth, about 80% of women experience an unexplained tearfulness. I had a big cry on the day of Hudson's birth when I woke up to find he'd been taken to the nursery and Bruce had gone home. I madly buzzed for help and the midwife said to me, 'What's up dear? You're not supposed to cry until day three.'

This is just the hormonal adjustment to breastfeeding and no longer being pregnant and it's OK for her to cry and be a sorry sack for a day or two. Don't try to be a bloke and solve her problems. Just let her be sad and tell her you love her. Tell her she's the most gorgeous woman on the planet and that she's even more beautiful with your baby in her arms.

If her sadness goes on for more than a few days, that's when you need to see your local doctor together to make sure she's not suffering from postnatal depression (PND).

According to Beyond Blue, an organisation working on the prevention and awareness of depression, PND affects almost 16% of new mothers. There are a number of factors that can contribute to the onset of PND, including a past history of depression, a stressful pregnancy, prolonged labour or difficult birth, lack of practical, financial or emotional support, difficulties with breastfeeding, sleep deprivation and having unrealistic expectations of motherhood.

Women who suffer from PND need to see a doctor and consider psychological treatment and/or medication to manage what is a treatable condition, but can sometimes be a serious issue for you and your family.

Make sure that your partner is well supported in these first days, weeks and months after your baby is born and take time to nurture your relationship. Help your partner find time to do things she enjoys other than caring for your new baby and spend time listening to your partner without feeling the need to solve all her problems and offer solutions. Don't take your partner's moodiness or irritability personally. It's not about you.

Sleep deprivation can be really tough in those first weeks. Make sure that you and your partner are each getting a total of 8 hours sleep every 24 hours. This might be four sleeps of two hours at a time, but aim for a total of eight hours in a day. You'll soon get used to napping whenever you can. In our house, sleep became currency. 'I'll clean the entire house if you let me sleep for two hours,' was a typical bargain when our kids were newborns.

In addition to lack of sleep, your partner may also be exhausted from the stress of adjusting to her new role. When she is stressed, her adrenal gland works overtime. Your job is to continue the role you played during the birth, making sure there are low levels of adrenalin in your partner's system. Help her to relax and stay calm. Fend off irritations and stresses wherever you can.

She also needs to avoid caffeine as this fires up the adrenal gland, which can be good in the short term, but in the long term will deplete her energy and hamper her immune system. Furthermore, caffeine in your partner's system will stimulate the baby via breast milk and will interfere with good sleeping patterns in your baby.

'When we are that exhausted, it's natural for the body to crave things that will give a quick fix, such as coffee and sugar,' says Chinese herbalist and acupuncturist, Naomi Abeshouse. 'It really is unfair that both of these things can work so well but for such a short time! Coffee will mess with your capacity to regulate your nervous system (and catch those important naps when you can during the day). Caffeine can also make you and your partner more edgy and anxious, which is unhelpful when you are already irritable with fatigue.

'Sugar will lead you on a cycle of ups and downs and not give you the sustained energy required for the task of caring for a newborn. Look out for the sneaky products that combine caffeine and sugar. Chocolate, unfortunately, is really not your friend at this time.'

It is very important that you help your partner to stay hydrated. She needs a lot of water while she is breastfeeding and recovering from the birth: about ten glasses a day and more in hot weather. This is very important. If your partner is dehydrated, she will be more tired and cranky, she'll have less milk to offer your baby and then your baby will be tired and cranky and then everyone's unhappy. Water, water, water! If your partner doesn't really like drinking water, add some lemon slices and fresh mint to make it more appetising.

> *I want to circumcise my sons but my wife is against it. What's the current thinking on this?*
>
> *There's nothing quite like circumcision to polarise opinions. Most men only prefer to circumcise their sons if they were circumcised themselves. 'Who needs the sleeping bag?' one dad said to me. Some believe that circumcision is important for religious reasons. However, since the 1970s, doctors have discouraged routine circumcision in infancy for a number of reasons. These days you have to go out of your way to request that your sons be circumcised. See the resources section for a good reference on circumcision and all the reasons why it is now avoided. Some circumcised dads are concerned that if they break the trend and don't circumcise their sons, they will look different and this could be a concern for boys. This is easily explained: Daddy looks different because he was born at a time when doctors thought it was a good idea to chop off the extra skin. When you were born, doctors had decided that it was better to leave it there.*

Low blood sugar levels will also make your partner tired and cranky. She needs small, nutritious meals often. Steer clear of soft drinks and other sugar-laden products. As author Michael Pollan[1] writes in his book *Food Rules*, 'Don't ingest foods made in places where everyone is required to wear a surgical cap. If it came from a plant, eat it; if it was made in a plant, don't.' This is my kind of no-fluff advice.

'If you are struggling to achieve a balanced diet for you and your partner, then consider supplements,' says Naomi Abeshouse. 'A good multivitamin and a quality fish oil are the bare basics for both of you. If she is feeling particularly weak, miserable or moody, consider seeing a Chinese herbalist for some herbs to help with this.'

After about three months, you and your partner will benefit from fitting some exercise into your lives. Don't put pressure on your partner to get fit and lose weight. Rather, emphasise that some exercise and fresh air will help her with her energy levels. Women who have just had a baby are very sensitive about their new body shape. I heaped on 26 kilos when I had my first child and I thought I was destined to be chubby forever. The weight did come off eventually – just in time to get pregnant with my second – but I truly thought I was going to be overweight forever and this was really upsetting.

Adelaide mother of seven, Helen Hriskin, says that her husband Romeo was instrumental in helping her not just to adjust to her new body but to admire it. 'About four months after the birth of the last of our brood of seven, I complained to Romeo that I was too fat and frumpy and couldn't fit into my clothes, not even my fat jeans!' says Helen. 'The best thing he's ever said to me was this: "Babe, you should be so proud of your body and the work it's done. You have grown seven beautiful babies to full term and birthed them all. That is so amazing and awe inspiring. I love you for you and I love all your bumps and lumps and battle scars!" What a wonderful man.'

Some exercise will certainly help your partner with her energy levels and the easiest solution for fitting exercise into your life is to put your baby in the pram and go for walks with your partner. Start with a 30-minute walk a few times a week and then build up to a 45-minute walk every day. Your energy levels will certainly benefit and so will your partner's self esteem. Most babies love a walk in the pram too.

Yoga is highly recommended for helping your partner bring her abdominal muscles back together and to strengthen her core and pelvic floor again. It will also give her a sanity break from baby duties and the feeding treadmill too. There are also 'mums and bubs' classes offered in most major cities where women can take their newborns to class and practice yoga with their baby on their yoga mat.

'Before practising yoga, women who have given birth should wait until the usual postnatal bleeding has completely stopped and they have

We'd like to consider environmentally responsible nappies for our baby. What are the options?

Your nappy choice is an important one. Nappies are changed 8-12 times a day for a newborn and 6-10 times a day as your baby grows. And it's not just the nappy to consider: it's also wipes, washing, disposal and convenience that all contribute to a nappy choice that is potentially costly to the environment. When it comes to considering the cost of nappies, disposable nappies cost more than $6000 per child compared to cloth nappies at around $1000, even when the cost of washing is factored in. The tide has turned towards cloth nappies. A Choice survey in the late 1990s showed that 85% of parents preferred disposable nappies while in 2010 only 60% prefer this option. Jannine Barron, founder of Australia's largest organic baby store, Nature's Child, offers a number of environmentally responsible nappy options. 'We want to support new parents with sustainable nappy solutions that suit their needs. Our cloth nappies are made from chemical-free bamboo or organic cotton using sustainable farming practices.' A mother of two herself, Jannine understands that the thought of using cloth nappies might be terrifying for some. 'Start with a few samples, try them and see what works for you. Have a clear intention before you start; this will keep you on track!' Following are nappy solutions that are both practical and environmentally friendly:

- Compostable disposable nappies
- Eco-disposables – fewer chemicals, no bleach
- Modern cloth nappies – cloth nappies in a pre-fitted shape that look like disposables but are made from cloth
- The classic, timeless towelling square nappy – fits all sizes, dries fast and presents the cheapest option. Some still think it's the best!

All nappy options and costs are listed in detail on the Nature's Child website at www.natureschild.com.au.

had their six week postnatal check up,' says Pam Sherwin, a Sydney yoga teacher specialising in prenatal and postnatal yoga.

'Women who have had a normal vaginal birth can start yoga once their baby is about six weeks old, as long as they have approval from their caregiver. Those who have had a Caesarean should wait at least 12 weeks and there should be no discomfort whatsoever when reaching arms above the head.'

Pam says that it is very important that your partner does not attempt sit ups or crunches until the abdominal muscles, which separate when a woman is pregnant, have come back together.

Make it easy for your partner to get to a weekly yoga class by taking your baby on a long bush walk in a baby backpack or doing several laps of your local park and meeting up afterwards so that your baby can have a feed. This way you're both getting some exercise.

At some point after the birth of your baby, your sex life will hopefully return. I am often asked when this will be. When? When? When? It really depends on your partner and how quickly she recovers from the birth and how exhausted she is in the first few months of motherhood. Some women have their sex drive back in action within three or four months but some take much longer.

To give you two examples from either end of the spectrum, a friend of mine says that when she left hospital after the birth of her second child, another boy, all she wanted to do was leap into bed with her husband to try for a girl. 'I can't believe how horny I was!' she told me. Emphasis in that example is on the *second child*. Recovery from birth is much quicker after subsequent babies.

Another friend of mine needed over a year before she could have sex with her husband again. For many women, sex is painful in the first months after giving birth and they need time to recover fully, especially if they have had an episiotomy.

Unfortunately it is common for women to find they lose spontaneous desire when they are dealing with the fatigue and stress of coping with young children. Sex therapist Bettina Arndt's book, *The Sex Diaries*, was based on ordinary couples keeping diaries about how they negotiate their sex supply. Many of Bettina's female diarists acknowledged that they lost interest in sex at this time in their lives.

Bettina's research showed that some women assume that if they don't feel like having sex, it just shouldn't happen. On the other hand, other women realise how important physical intimacy is to maintaining closeness in their relationship and make the effort to 'just do it', knowing that once they get started, they do enjoy the lovemaking.

Bettina quotes new research showing that many women can become aroused and reach orgasm without prior desire, provided they can get their head in the right place and let themselves enjoy the experience.

If you want your sex life back sooner rather than later, I've always thought it a good idea for fathers to do the housework. To my mind, there is nothing sexier than a man pushing a broom or folding laundry. It also means that your partner will have more energy for you at the end of the day.

Having said that, Bettina's research shows that this theory isn't always a winner. She had female diarists who said their husbands were 'domestic gods' but still got no sex. However, Bettina acknowledges that men who don't help around the house are unlikely to get much sex: 'Women whose husbands are lazy about sharing the chores are naturally likely to feel angry and resentful. Resentment is a huge passion-killer. Doing the laundry won't guarantee you get laid but not doing it may mean you haven't a chance,' she says.

There's also no reason why you can't be intimate without actually having penetrative sex. A good naked kiss and cuddle is still intimate.

Many men are interested to know whether sex will feel different after their partner has given birth. Some incorrectly assume that if a woman has had a Caesarean, she will suffer no pelvic floor damage at all, but this is not necessarily the case. The most common pelvic floor damage is caused when a woman carries her baby to full term, so women who have had a surgical delivery can still notice changes to their pelvic floor after the baby is born.

The fact is, your sex life *will* be different when it recommences after the birth. Throughout your partner's pregnancy, the hormone relaxin has been helping her body to prepare for the birth by softening the pubic bone. It softens everything else as well, so you may have noticed that sex with your partner felt different as her pregnancy progressed and her muscles loosened. Many men notice that after the birth, their partner actually feels tighter as relaxin is no longer loosening her joints and muscles.

One father told me how sex felt for him after the births of his children...

'We'd had a great sex life before the kids were born but it was more about quantity than quality, to be honest. Once we started a family, we were tired a lot of the time, especially my wife. It took us about six months after our first child was born before we were having sex again. It was fantastic! I had heard jokes from other men about sex after birth being like "throwing a sausage up the Grand Canyon" but that was rubbish. If anything, my wife felt tighter compared to sex when she was pregnant. We now have three kids and she had three vaginal births so I suppose there is some pelvic floor damage but I think sex is better since our babies were born. It's now about quality rather than quantity and my wife feels kind of collapsed inside. It's snugger, warmer and closer.'

You have a whole life of parenting ahead of you and there are other books to help you through that whole adventure. In the meantime, the best advice I can give you when it comes to parenting your child is to ignore advice! You know the kind I mean – the well-meaning, unsolicited and unprofessional advice that comes at you like a machine gun from family, friends and total strangers before and after you have a baby.

I really believe that you already have intuition as a parent and that you will work out what works best for you and your family. Having been involved in the birth, you have already created a special bond between you, your partner and your baby. Parenting is just building on that.

Work out what's best for your family and make the decision to ignore other people and their judgements. Having said that, make sure you don't judge other new parents and their choices. Wouldn't we have a happier world if nobody felt judged?

If you've just arrived home with your new baby but you read this chapter three months ago, these are the important points to remember:

- *Get your act together to bring your partner and baby home*
- *Arrange some extra home help around the house*
- *Manage visitors by putting your partner and baby first*
- *Make nappy changes your job, forever*
- *Keep an eye out for the baby blues*
- *Aim for eight hours sleep in any 24 hour period*
- *Make sure you are both getting good nutrition*
- *Try to work some exercise into your lives*
- *Take on the lion's share of housework if you're hoping for your sex life to resume*
- *Ignore unsolicited advice and go with what works for your family*

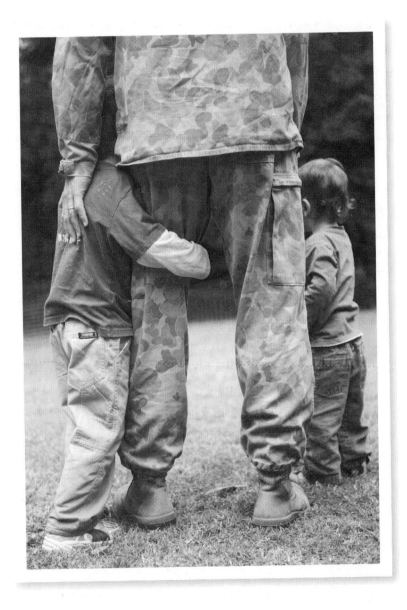

DAVID MAXWELL'S STORY

You bond with your baby when you change the nappies. I reckon a true man is a guy who'll do the housework.

Warrant Officer Class 1 David Maxwell* had always wanted to join the military. His grandfather had served in World War I and his father had been a World War II paratrooper in the British Army. After finishing school in Adelaide in 1985, David joined the army. He was based at Holsworthy before he did parachute training and was in the Red Beret Parachute Display Team with almost 200 jumps under his belt. David completed Special Forces selection and has been deployed to some of the world's worst trouble spots, including Iraq, East Timor, Sudan, Sinai and Bougainville. To the detriment of his army career, David has chosen to spend less time overseas and more time at home since his two sons were born, births after which he felt he needed a thorough military-style debriefing.

My father died when I was a baby. He died of a brain haemorrhage as a long-term result of a blunt force trauma inflicted when he was a prisoner of war in Poland. Before I was born, Mum had a premature baby, a girl, who died when she was three months old. After that Mum had a stillborn baby boy. I was her third child, who came out screaming, fit and strong, but my father died only three months after I was born. I'm told that my mother used to constantly prod me to make sure I was still alive.

This didn't pass on to me as anxiety for *my* children's health. I've seen the compatibility that my wife and I have as a strength and I have always applied this strength and confidence to our children. I have always felt confident that nothing would go wrong. As it turned out, the worst thing that happened at their births was that they both came out with cone heads!

I married a girl I met when I was on company exchange with the British Army and we settled in Brisbane. Unfortunately, the marriage didn't last. We had different life objectives, mine being the desire for children. I was young and not as understanding and sensitive as I could have been and overseas deployment can be very tough on a relationship.

About six months after my first marriage ended I got together with Sienna. We had one date and then I was deployed overseas, then went backpacking, so I didn't see her again for a long time. I had known Sienna for years – she was a civilian employee in the human resources department of the army. She knew what she was getting into, marrying a man in the armed services.

We'd been together for five years before we got engaged but we'd only been married for six weeks when Sienna fell pregnant. Calum came early so friends did the sums and thought we'd had a shotgun wedding but no, that wasn't the case.

I was excited as hell; I was the one doing the nesting, buying baby clothes and disinfecting everything. I made sure I was there for the births of my two boys. I was between deployments and had a twelve-month stint at home when Calum was born. Some army guys' wives have Caesareans because they can book in the date of the birth and make sure their partner is there for it, but we wanted a natural birth.

I wanted to do everything within my means to make the birth as comfortable as possible for my wife. If that meant going for a private obstetrician, that's what we had to do. Sienna wanted a female obstetrician and wanted to give birth as close to home as possible. There's a lot going on in a pregnant woman's body, so I wanted her to be as relaxed as she could be.

Sienna's waters broke three weeks early. I'd organised a golf game for that day and I had mates coming from the other side of town so I was kind of relieved when they told us that it was just a rupture of the membranes and the baby wouldn't necessarily arrive that day. I feel bad admitting to this, but Sienna let me have my round of golf and she stayed in hospital for another week before Calum was born.

Sienna's sister was with us for the birth. She's had four children and was there as the experienced female support. I felt quite comfortable with the whole birth process. I'd read the books. I was the theoretical expert! I gave her as much comfort as I could.

It wasn't a terribly long labour but when it came down to it, Calum got stuck and became distressed and the doctor had to use the vacuum to suck him out. Sienna also had to have an episiotomy but I didn't see any of that. She had said I wasn't allowed to go any lower than her waist. She didn't want me to have a different view of her 'down there' after the birth.

I've seen some horrendous situations on army deployments overseas – dead bodies, an horrific grenade incident, bodies fused together by fire. You're well prepared for it and have been trained to distance yourself from it. But when it came to childbirth and the woman I love, I really didn't want to see the war wounds my wife sustained through the birth, particularly the episiotomy. Not because it grossed me out but because it was happening to the woman I adore.

You can feel sympathy for your wife as she goes through childbirth but you can't feel empathy. As a man, you really have no idea how she is feeling.

Calum finally came out and was put straight onto Sienna's chest. He opened his eyes and he looked at me and that's when the tears welled up. The emotion just hit me and I stood there in disbelief. There he was, after all these years. I had to go into the toilet and console myself, man myself up a bit. I hadn't expected to cry.

Calum is something between Sienna and me that is completely

unique. We produced something so beautiful.

Within thirty seconds of being born, Calum did a poo on Sienna, which was better out than in, if you ask me!

When army personnel are deployed overseas, they receive quite detailed psychological briefings and debriefings. It sounds callous, but I felt like I needed a debrief after the births more than I had after my deployments overseas.

I took a lot of time off work to be home with Sienna and Calum. Most people don't realise that the army is really flexible and very family friendly. They'll do all they can to support you, especially with the first child. I was entitled to two weeks of paternity leave, which can be used anytime in the first twelve months after your baby is born. I added another two weeks of annual leave so that I could be home for a whole month, then six months later I took another few weeks off to give Sienna a break.

Having a newborn at home seemed worse than any deployment or war zone I've ever been to! I like my sleep. Deployments are for a fixed time but the challenges of a baby go on for years. Sienna's one of these people who can survive on five or six hours sleep a night. She was also adjusting to broken sleep when she was pregnant so when Calum arrived, she was already used to it. She breastfed for about a month but this was a struggle because Calum didn't latch on properly. After a month we switched to bottle-feeding and I did the weekend night feeds.

Calum was about two and a half when Sienna fell pregnant with Owen. She craved Homer Hudson ice cream so I was buying about five tubs every week. The strange thing was, I craved the same foods as she did.

Owen was a big eight-pound boofer when he was born and after his due date, had been getting bigger by the day, so two weeks after the due date Sienna was induced. It was a much longer labour than Calum's.

I tried to be supportive but I made a really dumb comment. Just when she was about to start pushing, I said, 'The hard part's all over!' and the room went silent. What I should have said was that the end was in sight. 'What do you mean the hard part's over?' she shouted at me. At least it distracted her for the time being.

After a long labour, Sienna was fully dilated and ready to push but Owen got stuck, just as his brother had and Sienna was prepped up and wheeled in for a Caesarean. The midwife was convinced that Sienna could do it naturally but the obstetrician still arranged for the Caesar. Next thing we know, Sienna's in an operating theatre surrounded by about 12 medical staff. At the last minute, the doctor said, 'Just give me one more try to get this baby out,' and he got out the vacuum.

Out Owen came! He was born naturally and the Caesarean was avoided.

The whole thing was exhausting; we'd been going all night. I sat down once the birth was over and they asked if I wanted to cut the umbilical cord. I said, 'Holy crap, I can hardly stand.'

I noticed that they distracted me from the damage repair for Sienna and the midwife ushered me over to look after the baby. Sienna had to go to recovery and I took Owen to the ward and it felt like it took forever for her to come back to us.

We had to share a room with another mother after Owen's birth, which wasn't so good. Sienna was self-conscious about having people she didn't know walking through our room. For the same reason, it took Sienna about three months before she was willing to breastfeed in public. After a couple of days we were given our own room and could really begin bonding with Owen without interruption. After some of the hospitals I have seen overseas with 35 mothers in one ward, we're very lucky in Australia, but a room to ourselves made a big difference to our privacy and getting enough rest.

You get a lot of advice when you're having a baby and we tried to absorb the best ideas from everybody. One of those ideas was to have a present from the baby for his older brother – a helicopter (wocka-wocka as he calls it).

Sienna is such a natural mother and I've always had confidence in her. I look at her now in a more mature way: she's the mother of my children. Now we have two children and we're a little older, we've been through a bit of a re-exploration of each other and our sex life, especially now that Sienna isn't so tired all the time. It's a whole new phase in our life together.

Even though I never had a father – I was raised by my mother and my nan – I knew I had a good temperament for fatherhood. A mate of mine told me about ten years ago that he thought I would be a good dad and I've always remembered that.

I craved children for nearly a decade so when it came down to it, I was prepared to change the nappies and give Sienna time to herself. You bond with your baby when you change the nappies. It gives you the freedom to spend time alone with them. I reckon a true man is a guy who'll do the housework. I've also learned what not to do from observing some other fathers who distance themselves from their children.

I think anyone who really wants children will be a natural parent, provided they're not selfish. My mum made huge sacrifices for me and I'm willing to do that for my kids.

* Names have been changed according to Australian Army protocol.

CHAPTER 16

BREASTFEEDING FOR BLOKES

Breastfeeding is a tricky department and your partner will need support from you to get this important part of mothering underway smoothly. It can also be a touchy subject and some mothers feel upset or guilty if they don't or can't breastfeed their baby. Your partner might need some extra love and support if that happens.

The World Health Organisation recommendation is for babies to be exclusively breastfed for the first six months of their lives. There is overwhelming evidence and enormous health marketing oomph behind the importance of breast milk. However, if a woman is suffering from constant, crippling bouts of mastitis or has a very low milk supply, this advice can be tough to take.

Most mothers in Australia start by breastfeeding their baby. It's something that babies and mums are made to do, but it's not always easy. The best thing you can do is to help your partner establish and maintain breastfeeding and if she just can't pull it off, help her feel confident that she's done the best she can, that she's still a great mother. You can remind her that breastfeeding is not the benchmark of quality motherhood, but simply a health recommendation.

Research shows that a woman is more likely to breastfeed and for longer if she has the support of a partner who knows what he's doing and is engaged in the process. So read on.

Professional help

Most Australian hospitals have professional lactation consultants available who can help your partner start the breastfeeding process with confidence. If your baby is born in hospital, make the most of these in-house services while your partner and baby are there. If your baby is feeding comfortably before leaving hospital, then your partner is more likely to be confident and less likely to have problems once you are at home.

If your partner does have breastfeeding problems, encourage her to seek professional help promptly. That's the key: get help quickly! It's no use struggling for weeks when you can access professional assistance by contacting the hospital again, or looking for a private lactation consultant in your area, or by a call to the free Australian Breastfeeding Association Helpline (see page 256 for ABA contact details).

The women on the ABA helpline are experienced breastfeeding counsellors who take calls from home. They are mothers themselves and they understand what your partner is going through. They really are angels.

Dads can call the breastfeeding helpline as well if they are worried about any breastfeeding issues. Sometimes some reassurance is all you need so that you know things are going normally.

Sore nipples can be a challenge during the early days. For most women there is some soreness as their nipples adjust to all this new attention from their baby. For some women, the nipples can crack and bleed and become very painful indeed.

Problems like this can be minimised if your partner has good advice early on to make sure your baby is breastfeeding well. At any time, if your partner is in pain and her nipples are sore or bleeding, it's important to get good help, fast.

Some babies may have physical problems such as tongue-tie that will mean they don't breastfeed well and may hurt their mother's nipples. Have your baby checked by a breastfeeding professional to rule this out and make sure your partner gets help to be sure that your baby is positioned well. These simple things can make the difference between breastfeeding being easy or very difficult.

One of the best remedies for sore nipples is breast milk. It's magic stuff. After a feed, your partner can squeeze some milk out of her nipple and gently wipe it all over the whole areola then allow it to be absorbed before clipping up her maternity bra.

Pure lanolin works well for soothing sore, cracked nipples but it may leave an oily stain on clothes so your partner may like to use some breast pads to protect her bras and T-shirts.

If your partner is in a lot of pain, even after help from a lactation consultant, a silicon nipple guard may work well for her.

It will be your job to provide all these items. You should be the one beating a path to the chemist in the first few weeks after the birth, not your partner!

The breastfeeding trifecta

The beginning of the breastfeeding process is a time of learning for mother and baby. Making sure that your partner has encouragement, support and access to help in the first six weeks is important. Eating well, resting often and feeding when your baby needs to, will all help build a good milk supply and a confident mother.

Midwife Akal Khalsa says that the three most important things to remember for building a healthy milk supply are diet, fluids and rest.

Breastfeeding mums don't need a special diet; just a healthy, balanced one. Fresh fruits and vegetables, with protein from whatever sources you usually eat (either meat or vegetarian alternatives) will help to keep mother and baby healthy. Your partner may be hungrier while breastfeeding, so adding regular healthy snacks during the day will keep her energy levels at their best.

Breastfeeding mothers need to drink several glasses of water a day. When your partner sits down to feed your baby, give her a glass of water to drink while she feeds.

Some herbal teas, including chamomile and fennel, are said to support healthy lactation. Drinking herbal teas will also help your partner's water intake and help her avoid dehydration.

Another important change to consider for your family's diet is to cut out junk food. Chips, chocolate, biscuits and cakes will not help build your partner's milk supply.

'Eliminate junk food entirely!' says Akal. 'Junk food contains nothing but empty calories. It will not give your partner any nutritional benefit and will in fact deplete the B vitamins that would otherwise be used to maintain a healthy nervous system.'

Become the hardware specialist

At some later stage your partner may consider returning to work or you may just like to have a babysitter or grandparent look after the baby so that you can have a night out together. This will require expressing milk and storing it so that your baby can be fed in your partner's absence – opening up a whole new area of hardware for you.

Expressing milk for an occasional or weekly night out is easy with a good quality hand-operated breast pump. Milk can be collected over a couple of days and your baby will only need 100 – 120ml for a feed.

Your partner returning to work might mean expressing every day, so a good electric pump will really help. These often come in kits with a cooler bag especially for the job. If you only need it for a few weeks, hiring may be the go. See the resources section for places to buy or hire.

You will also need bottles, silicon teats, a bottle brush and a steriliser to keep it all clean, as well as freezer bags in which to store the milk. As I said, lots of hardware and a few hundred dollars worth of gear to invest in, but it will be worth it.

Some babies' bottle brands are made from polycarbonate, the evil plastic that contains BPA or Bisphenol A. This chemical leaches into the liquid you're feeding your baby, mimicking oestrogen. Research has made links between this chemical and breast cancer. Babies bottles made from polycarbonate are being phased out by retailers in Australia but have not been banned outright (as they have been in Europe and Canada). Be sure to only buy bottles for your baby that are labelled 'BPA free'.

This information is also important to remember when your child is older. Avoid plastic water bottles that have the recycle code number seven (which includes polycarbonates) imprinted on the bottom. Bottles that have a recycle code number one are typically the plastic bottles that spring water products are sold in and they should be used only once and thrown away. Look for water bottles that are clearly labelled 'BPA-free' for your kids.

The best babies' bottle sterilisers are the kind you can put in the microwave with some added water. You can sterilise your bottles in a large pot on the stove but many a baby's bottle has been fried beyond recognition when the pot has been forgotten.

You need to take care in labelling the breast milk and freezing it correctly, throwing out any that has passed its use-by date. Your breast milk bags will come with instructions on how to store the milk correctly.

Never heat breast milk in the microwave as this can destroy the nutritional content and microwaves are prone to overheating. You can buy bottle warmers that heat the bottle in a small amount of hot water. Alternatively, you can rest the bottle in a bowl of hot water for about five minutes. Shake it gently, then test the milk on your inner wrist to make sure it is not too hot for your baby.

Keep an eye out

When your partner is breastfeeding, her breasts will become much bigger. MUCH bigger! You might think the engorgement of her bust is a great new development but it can be painful for her. When her breasts are sore and hard, your partner needs either to feed the baby or express the milk to relieve the pressure. Behave yourself or she might squirt you in the eye!

Mastitis is an inflammation of the breast, which can be very painful. Feeding often and starting each feed on the opposite side to the start of the last feed can help to keep breasts from becoming inflamed. This is because the baby usually sucks harder on the first breast.

If your partner develops mastitis, she will be encouraged to keep on breastfeeding. The milk is still fine for your baby and the problem clears up faster when the breasts are emptied often. Some women need antibiotics so that the problem doesn't worsen. If your partner has red, sore breasts and a fever, or has aching joints, it's best to get some medical help right away.

Non-infective mastitis is sometimes treated with cabbage leaves. Believe it or not, a cabbage leaf tucked inside your partner's bra will cool down the breast and as her body heats the leaf, it releases various anti-inflammatory chemicals. A cabbage leaf is also the perfect shape to cup a sore bosom. Add a cabbage to your shopping list.

Your partner should change feeding positions now and then to make sure she is draining all the milk ducts. According to Akal, if your partner has a blockage in the breast she should feed with the baby's chin pointing towards the blockage. This makes the most of the baby's strongest sucking power, applied in the right direction.

A breastfeeding pillow is a useful item to buy for your partner so that she can lay the baby across the pillow on her lap and relax while feeding.

Consider a compromise

Sometimes mothers have problems that mean they can't breastfeed sufficiently for some or all of their baby's needs. If this is the case for you and your partner, consider mixed feeding before ruling out breastfeeding altogether. This means giving your baby some formula as well as breastfeeding.

A lactation consultant can help you make a feeding plan to get the most from breastfeeding, even if you need to include infant formula as well. Stopping breastfeeding suddenly can cause problems for your partner and baby, so help from a health professional is really important.

If you decide to include formula in your baby's diet, all the above sterilising information and equipment still applies.

There is a lot to the art of breastfeeding and this chapter can't cover it all. Instead I have focused on the areas in which you can best support your partner. Remember, women who have a supportive and knowledgeable partner are more likely to breastfeed and for longer than those who don't.

The important breastfeeding tips to remember are:

- *Get some professional help pronto if your partner has problems*
- *Remember the trifecta of breastfeeding needs: good diet, plenty of water and enough rest*
- *Become the hardware specialist when it comes to all the gear involved with expressing milk, storing it and bottle feeding*
- *Keep an eye out for mastitis and if it appears to be infective mastitis, get some medical attention quickly*
- *If problems persist, consider mixed feeding with infant formula before ruling out breastfeeding altogether*

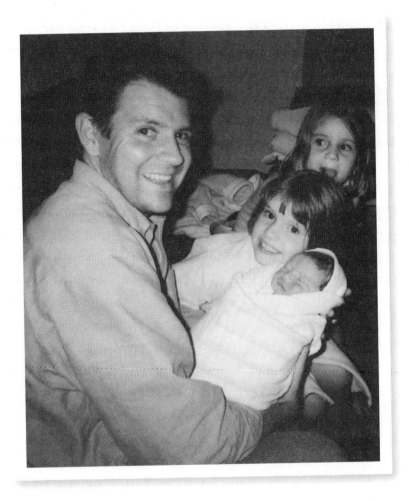

MIKE BAIRD'S STORY

I had an incredible sense of awe and respect for what Kerryn had achieved. There's a moment where you just think, 'My wife has turned into Mohammad Ali!'

Mike Baird grew up surfing the northern beaches of Sydney. With an economics arts degree, he began a career in banking and was appointed Account Manager in Corporate Banking and Finance within the National Australia Bank at the ripe old age of 23. He moved quickly up the ranks within NAB, including a long stint in London where he was Head of Originations, UK and Europe. In his late twenties, Mike headed in a new direction and studied in Canada to become a minister. When he and wife Kerryn learned that they were expecting their first child, Mike rethought his future, deciding that with his specific skills, a career in politics might well allow him to make a wider contribution to his community than a future in the clergy. The Bairds came back to Australia and Mike worked for Deutsche Bank and finally HSBC. Then, after 18 years in banking, Mike followed his father's footsteps into politics and was elected State Member for Manly in 2007, at the same time as his father was the Federal Member for Cook. Mike was appointed to the front bench of the NSW Coalition and managed various portfolios before being promoted to the role of Shadow Treasurer. He is widely tipped as a strong contender for future Premier of New South Wales. Here he tells the stories of the births of his children with spine-tingling clarity and honest admissions in terms of his own shortcomings.

My wife and I were married for about seven years before we started a family. The first time that the idea of having a baby became real for me was when I was studying at Bible College in Canada and I had a call from one of my best mates, to say his wife was pregnant. My best mate was going to have a baby and the joy in his emails and in his voice was very apparent. It brought home to me that one day that would happen for us.

We started talking about having a baby and then we started trying to conceive and a few months later we were doing a mad dash around Vancouver to find a pharmacy open to buy a pregnancy test. It was a wild mixture of panic and excitement. We were in shock when we saw the little pink line.

It all went well from there. We saw an obstetrician in Canada but then came home to Sydney to have our baby. I'll never forget hearing our baby's heartbeat at the first ultrasound. It was an emotional time for both of us.

Kerryn and I were really excited as the birth approached. I went along to the antenatal classes where all the blokes seemed slightly bewildered. They asked us guys what we were thinking about it all and one brave guy put his hand up and said, 'I really like my wife's big breasts!' That kind of broke the ice.

We had Laura at Manly hospital. During the labour I did my best to help: turning on the shower when Kerryn needed it, massaging her back, holding her hand, but I kind of felt like someone else was running a marathon and I was just on the side lines clapping.

There was one moment when I went to get some water for Kerryn and checked the cricket scores on the way. She's never forgotten it and still holds that against me! It was Australia vs New Zealand, by the way.

Right at the end of labour, during transition, Kerryn was in intense pain. She asked for an epidural but the midwives said it was too late to have one. Kerryn didn't lose control but I was starting to worry about how much pain she was in. In the end she used some gas and that got her through the worst of it.

I had an incredible sense of awe and respect for what Kerryn had achieved. There was a moment where I thought, 'My wife has turned into Mohammad Ali!' She was just incredible.

I watched our baby come out and it was a wonderful combination of complete chaos and exhilaration. It was almost a spiritual experience seeing new life being born. Out of chaos and mess came this beautiful new life that we had created.

When I held Laura in my arms for the first time I couldn't believe how perfect she was. Her cheeks, her nose, her little fingers were just perfect.

Kerryn bounced back really well in the hours after the birth. She was buzzing. She looked great.

Something that I regret is that after Laura was born, I took only a week off work. I was very busy, working round the clock and when I look back, I should have been much more supportive. I have no doubt that my absence was a contributing factor to the postnatal depression that Kerryn developed. I feel really crap about that.

We weren't at all prepared for life after the birth. Laura was a really good baby but Kerryn had trouble breastfeeding. We hadn't prepared for breastfeeding because we just didn't think it would be an issue. There was one night when we were up at 3am and Kerryn described the pain of breastfeeding like a knife stabbing her in the breast. We had a breast pump going but she was in agony. No one had warned us about that.

I would tell any expectant dad to prepare well for *after the birth*. You only get that time with your baby once. I should have stopped everything I was doing and given all my support to Kerryn as my number one priority instead of focusing on work. I suppose I had a distorted perspective. I'd like to kid myself that it was driven by the need to provide for my new family, but ultimately I've realised it was pretty self-centred. Work was my identity and I thought that the transaction I was working on was the most important thing in the world when ten kilometres away, my wife was at home in incredible need. It's taken me a while to wise up to that.

Cate's birth was a lot more dramatic. There had been talk about relocating overseas for work and then right at the end of the pregnancy it was confirmed that we were off to London. That took focus away from the birth but we knew what we were in for this time, or so we thought.

The labour took a long time to get established so Kerryn was induced with a drip and her waters were broken. It went well but she was in lots of pain. I did my best to help. Once Cate was born, I held her in my arms and I was even more overwhelmed than I had been when Laura was born. I think that's because Laura was now a little two year old running around and I could remember when she looked just like this little newborn.

Very soon after the birth, I noticed that Kerryn didn't look so great. She was pale and quiet. She was having some dinner when she said, 'I think I'm bleeding.'

Before we knew it, the midwife confirmed that Kerryn was having a ferocious postpartum haemorrhage. One minute there we were quietly with our baby and next thing it seemed like there were about twenty people in the room with lights and a sense of controlled panic.

Kerryn lost consciousness and there was blood everywhere. At that moment, I looked at her and I wasn't sure, but I thought she might have died. I didn't know what to think. I held Cate in my arms and looked at her, thinking that she would never know her beautiful mum. They were the darkest moments of my life.

The two midwives on duty that night, Emma and Ann, saved Kerryn's life. She had to have a blood transfusion and she was in hospital for a couple of weeks with a much longer recovery time than the first birth. I will always be in debt to those midwives who worked so hard to save Kerryn.

Now I look at my wife and every day is special. My perspective that work was the centre of my life was completely smashed that night.

I think the trauma of that birth had something to do with Kerryn's postnatal depression after Cate was born. I don't want to give myself too much credit but I think I was more aware and able to support Kerryn better after Cate was born than I had been after the birth of our first little girl.

We hadn't planned to have three kids. Our son was a little surprise. Kerryn said to me on the phone, 'If I had some exciting news, should I tell you in person or on the phone?' I said 'You're pregnant!' and she said, 'YES!'

The obstetrician for Luke's birth had it all mapped out so that any bleeding could be controlled. This meant having an epidural and a low dose drip to manage the contractions. We had a lot of confidence in her as our obstetrician. She had to flick Luke around because he was in a posterior position and she did that brilliantly.

The labour was about seven hours long but nothing like the turbo-charged labour of the previous birth.

I didn't like the thought of the epidural going in but once it was all set up I watched the contractions on the monitor and as they got stronger and stronger and Kerryn wasn't reacting in any way to the pain, I became a big believer in epidurals!

With Lukie, the war wounds of the last two had prepared us well for having our third. He's four years younger than Cate so the girls were old enough to entertain themselves and Kerryn coped incredibly well.

Kerryn and I are as in love today as we were when we were first together but we've been through a lot since then. It would be fair to say that supporting Kerryn through the births of our babies and the months thereafter has forced me to grow up, to rethink my priorities and to man-up to the task of fatherhood.

AFTERWORD

Good luck. If you've read all the way to the end of this book, something tells me you're going to be a really good support partner and a fabulous dad.

I love receiving emails from the men who attend our Beer + Bubs sessions at the pub to tell me how their births went. I have a soft spot for the boys' experiences. So please email me and tell me how the birth went for you, what it felt like to become a father and how you supported your partner. What worked? What was a disaster? How did it *feel*? I'd love to know. Email me via the website at *www.beerandbubs.com.au*

Love Lucy

RESOURCES

Baby essentials

Nature's Child is Australia's largest online organic baby store (with a retail store in Byron Bay) chock-full of environmentally friendly essentials including the best baby's bottom balm in the whole world. *www.natureschild.com.au*

Breastfeeding helpline

Call the Australian Breastfeeding Association's 24 hour helpline if you need some assistance. They'll even give fathers some coaching on how to help their partner with breastfeeding problems. Phone 1800 686 268. *www.breastfeeding.asn.au*

Circumcision

If you're undecided about whether to opt for circumcision for your son, visit this website for information. *www.circinfo.org*

Depression prevention and treatment

These websites are useful resources on depression for mums and dads. The Black Dog Institute site includes a self test for postnatal depression. *www.blackdoginstitute.com.au* and *www.beyondblue.org.au*

Fatherhood resources

Visit these Australian websites for free access to parenting articles specifically for fathers, as well as other resources. *www.fatherhood.org.au* and *www.fatherhood.net.au*

Find a doula
This is Australia's largest online directory of doulas or childbirth attendants from Hobart to Cairns, Sydney to Perth. The website is free for couples to use to find a doula to support them before and after the birth and they can post feedback about their doula afterwards.
www.findadoula.com.au

Good Beginnings
Good Beginnings provides community-supported early intervention programs for children and their families including dads' programs, advice and information for parents.
www.goodbeginnings.net.au

Head to the pub in the name of childbirth
If you've enjoyed reading this book, you'd enjoy a Beer + Bubs session at the pub. Expectant fathers have the opportunity to ask the questions they may not want to ask in hospital antenatal classes and can meet other dads in the same boat. Visit the website for dates and venues around Australia.
www.beerandbubs.com.au

Hardware: Breastfeeding
For all the bits and bobs to support breastfeeding, visit the Australian Breastfeeding Association's online store. There are also ABA retail stores in Melbourne and Brisbane.
www.mothersdirect.com.au

Heat packs
To buy the heat packs I recommend, visit the Remo website and search for Shin Bio Heat Packs. Remo delivers all over Australia.
www.remogeneralstore.com.au

Men's Line Australia

Men's Line offers free 24 Hour phone support for all men, including fathers. Phone 1300 78 99 78. The Men's Line website also has a document library of useful information, articles, reports and fact sheets specifically written for men and fathers.

www.menslineaus.org.au

Network with other dads

This is an online resource for both new and experienced fathers. It includes parenting articles and a forum for linking up with other dads.

www.dadsclub.com.au

Pregnancy Support Hotline

This free 24 hour support hotline could be very helpful to you if your partner is really struggling with her pregnancy. Phone 1300 139 313.

www.pregnancysupport.com.au

SIDS and Kids

Make it a priority to know the facts about preventing Sudden Infant Death Syndrome. Research into this syndrome and awareness of the ways to prevent it has reduced deaths in Australia from over 500 per year in the 1980s to fewer than 140 in 2000. Visit the SIDS website and click on 'safe sleeping' for further details on the strategies to prevent SIDs in your household.

www.sidsandkids.org

Standards for baby products

Find out what to look for in terms of safety when buying baby products including child restraint rules and guidelines for cots, prams and high chairs. Visit the Fair Trading website and search for 'baby products'.

www.fairtrading.nsw.gov.au

RECOMMENDED READING

Australian Baby Guide

The Australian Baby Guide is a comprehensive online resource brimming with expert articles, reassuring parenting advice, a reputable directory of products and services and an online forum to connect with other parents and professionals.

www.australianbabyguide.com.au

Baby Love **by Robin Barker**

This 700-page whopper is like the instruction manual that didn't come with your baby. There's no need to read it from cover to cover, just use it as a reference book and look up things as they happen. Robin takes a balanced view of how to care for your new family member.

www.panmacmillan.com.au

Birth Right **by Susan Ross**

If you are right at the beginning of the pregnancy roller coaster, this is an excellent book for helping you decide what care model will suit you: public hospital, private obstetrician or homebirth? When I'm Prime Minister, all couples will be given this book by their GP when their positive pregnancy test is confirmed!

www.birthright.com.au

Breastfeeding Naturally **by the Australian Breastfeeding Assoc.**

This book is the most comprehensive guide to breastfeeding in Australia. Subscribe to the ABA and receive a free copy.

www.mothersdirect.com.au

Manhood by Steve Biddulph

Every man should read this book whether he's a father or not. Over 150,000 other men can't be wrong! In *Manhood*, Biddulph tackles two important things for men: creating a healthy masculinity, and how men can free themselves from outdated roles. If you've read *Manhood* before, now is a good time to reread it as you become a father for the first time. *www.finch.com.au*

Pregnancy Loss: Surviving Miscarriage and Stillbirth by Zoe Taylor

This book is the first complete Australian resource written to provide parents with information and guidance to support them through the grieving process after miscarriage or stillbirth. A percentage of profits from the sale of this book goes to the Stillbirth Foundation Australia. *www.pregnancylossbook.com*

The Sex Diaries by Bettina Arndt

If you really want to understand what's going on in your partner's head when it comes to sex, read this book. Sex therapist and clinical psychologist Bettina Arndt studied 98 couples to work out why most men want more sex than their female partners and how this can be negotiated to sustain loving relationships. It's not a heavy research paper, it's a great read and Bettina's writing style is highly entertaining. *www.bettinaarndt.com.au*

Sleeping Like a Baby by Pinky McKay

This book is full of simple sleep solutions for infants and toddlers, based on a natural, intuitive approach to settling your child. Pinky is a certified lactation consultant, infant massage instructor and runs baby sleep seminars in and around Melbourne, as well as online seminars for those who live elsewhere around the country. *www.pinkymckay.com.au*

ACKNOWLEDGEMENTS

Producing this book was like one of my pregnancies – nine months of hard slog with lots of people supporting me along the way, then something I'm very proud of at the end. I would like to thank the following people for their help:

The fabulous fathers who shared their personal stories in the pages of this book – thank you for sharing the kind of insight that only a father in the trenches of parenthood can offer. Most of you had never heard of me before I came asking for an interview, so thank you for trusting me with your story and lending this book a little of your well-earned high profile. Thank you Jud Arthur, Mike Baird, Mark Ferguson, David Galilee, Danny Green, Gerrard Gosens, Digby Hone, David Maxwell, Mark Occhilupo, Paul Osborne, Adam Spencer, Paul Treseder, Charlie Teo, James Tomkins and Tim Vincent.

The health professionals who have given this book the medical authenticity it deserves – thank you for being so generous with your time and expertise: obstetrician and gynaecologist Dr John Keogh, obstetrician and fertility specialist Dr Ric Porter, obstetrician and gynaecologist Dr Gary Sykes, Chinese herbalist Naomi Abeshouse, midwife Akal Khalsa, sex therapist Bettina Arndt, birth consultant Denise Love, Associate Professor of Midwifery Hannah Dahlen, yoga teacher Pam Sherwin and aromatherapist Vickie Hingston-Jones.

Rosemary Schaffler – my editor and Mum. Thank you for slaving over every page in this book to knock it into shape, taking a good concept and helping to make it into something really fantastic. Thank you also for slaving over me: giving birth to me in the first place, teaching me to write, expecting nothing but the best and nurturing the mother in me.

Akal Khalsa – our midwife who cared for me through the pregnancies and births of our two girls with such love and then consulted in a professional capacity on this book with such attention to detail.

Sally Macarthur – for your valuable input. As a published academic author, your belief in my book concept has been such a blessing.

The team of doers who assisted with proof reading and valuable content contributions – Katrina McKinnon, Julia Thomas, Zoe Taylor, Michelle Galilee, Jane Lawrence, Davinia Jones and Marija Sprem.

Jannine Barron, Nature's Child – for hosting the first pregnancy retreat in Byron Bay and showing me that childbirth could be one of the best days in your life, then seven years later, believing in this book!

Adam Dipper – my side kick and graphic designer at Pure Graphics during this project, for putting up with more talk about childbirth than your average childless man in his early twenties should have to bear.

Lisa Messenger and Claire Livingston at the Messenger Group – for seeing that this book was a winner and helping me get it off the ground.

The friends and family who let me publish their personal experiences and words of wisdom throughout this book – thanks for sharing (in no particular order): Justine Cooper, Melinda Crocker, Sharon Geyer, Fiona McManus, Fiona Ross, Jessica Duffy, Davinia Jones, Leon Travis, Mika and Peter Richardson, Michael and Rebecca Schaffler, Peter and Kara Schaffler, Emily and Ben Board, Helen and Romeo Hriskin, Nic Arthur, Sue and Graeme Inglis, Jane Lawrence, Darren McMahon, Barry and Andrea Jacobs and all the wonderful couples I have supported over the years whose stories pepper this book with reality.

Bruce Perry – I picked a winner when I married Bruce. Some people have asked if I was inspired to create the pub workshops because I was let down by him when I gave birth. This isn't the case at all – quite the opposite. He was an amazing support through my three labours, supported me to develop Beer + Bubs and then to write this book. He's a good man and a wonderful father. Thank you Bruce.

NOTES

Chapter 1: The expectant father's job description

1. Odent, Michel MD. Midwifery, *Is the Participation of the Father at Birth Dangerous?*, Today Issue 51, Autumn 1999.

2. Odent, Michel MD, *A top obstetrician on why men should NEVER be at the birth of their child*, Daily Mail, 15 April 2006.

Chapter 2: Call for reinforcements

1. Klaus, M.H., Kennell, J. H., Klaus, P.H., *The Doula Book: How a trained labour companion can help you have a shorter, easier and healthier birth.* Second Edition. Perseus Publishing, 2002.

Chapter 4: Understanding labour pain

1. Hirsh, Adam T., George, Steven Z., Bialosky, Joel E. and Robinson, Michael E. *Fear of Pain, Pain Catastrophizing, and Acute Pain Perception: Relative Prediction and Timing of Assessment.* Published in final edited form as: J Pain. 2008 September; 9(9): 806–812. Published online 2008 May 16. doi: 10.1016/j.jpain.2008.03.012.

2. Jackson, Todd et al., *Gender differences in pain perception: the mediating role of self-efficacy beliefs.* Sex Roles: A Journal of Research, December 2002.

3. Liem, Edwin B., M.D., Joiner, Teresa V., B.S.N., Tsueda, Kentaro, M.D. and Sessler, Daniel I., M.D., *Increased Sensitivity to Thermal Pain and Reduced Subcutaneous Lidocaine Efficacy in Redheads.* Published in final edited form as: Anesthesiology. 2005 March; 102(3): 509–514.

4. Kariminia, Azar, Chamberlain, Marie E, Keogh, John and Shea, Agnes, *Randomised controlled trial of effect of hands and knees posturing on incidence of occiput posterior position at birth.*

Chapter 5: Practical ideas for pain management

1. Anim-Somuah M, Smyth RMD, Howell C.J et al., *Epidural versus non-epidural or no analgesia in labour.* 2005. Cochrane Database of Systematic Reviews Issue 4. Art no CD000331.

Chapter 6: Supporting your partner through loss

1. Stanton C, Lawn J, Rahman H, Wilczynska-Ketende K, Hill K. *Stillbirth rates: delivering estimates in 190 countries. Lancet 2006; 367: 1489-94.*

Chapter 8: Prelabour

1. Simkins, Penny, *The Birth Partner: Everything you need to know to help a woman through childbirth,* Second Edition, Harvard Common Press, 2001.

Chapter 12: Third stage of labour

1. Chaparro, C.M., Neufeld, L.M, Tena, Alavez G, Eguia-Liz, Cedillo R, Dewey, K.G, *Effect of timing of umbilical cord clamping on iron status in Mexican infants: a randomised controlled trial.* Lancet 2006; 367: 1997–2004.
2. *Rocking the Cradle – A Report into Childbirth Procedures,* Commonwealth of Australia Senate Report, December 1999.

Chapter 13: After the birth: the first few hours

1. Odent, Michel, *The Scientification of Love,* Free Association Books, 1999.

Chapter 15: Life after birth

1. Pollan, Michael, *Food Rules: an Eater's Manual,* Penguin Books, 2010.

BIBLIOGRAPHY

Arndt, Bettina, *The Sex Diaries*, Melbourne University Press, 2009.

Balaskas, Janet, *The Water Birth Book*, Thorsons, 2004.

Commonwealth of Australia Senate Report, *Rocking the Cradle – A Report into Childbirth Procedures*, December 1999.

Green, Danny with Lane, Daniel, *Closed Fists, Open Heart: the Danny Green Story*, ABC Books, 2008.

Occhilupo, Mark and Baker, Tim, *Occy: The Rise and Fall and Rise of Mark Occhilupo*, Ebury Press, 2008.

Odent, Michel, *The Scientification of Love*, Revised edition, Free Association Books, 2001.

Simkins, Penny, *The Birth Partner: Everything you need to know to help a woman through childbirth*, Second Edition, Harvard Common Press, 2001.

Pollan, Michael, *Food Rules: An Eater's Manual*, Penguin Books, 2010.

Wyndham, Susan, *Life In His Hands*, Picador, 2008.

Klaus, Marshall, Kennell, John and Klaus, Phyllis, *The Doula Book: How a trained labor companion can help you have a shorter, easier and healthier birth*, Second Edition, Perseus Books Group, 2002.

INDEX

Abeshouse, Naomi, 64, 226-227

acupressure, 64, 65

acupuncture, 20, 67

adrenalin, 4, 68-9, 114-5, 117, 133, 146, 162, 200, 226

advocacy, 111-7

after birth pains, 96, 198-9

afterbirth, *see* placenta

amniotic fluid, 22, 63, 131

anaesthetic: general, 208-9, 212; local, 87, 185; spinal block 208

antenatal classes, 6, 60, 113, 146

Arndt, Bettina, 231

aromatherapy, 80-1, 89, 134, 143

Arthur, Jud, 203-6

baby blues, 96, 224, 233, *see also* post natal depression,

baby: at the moment of birth, 175; bathing, 199-200, 224; caring for, 222-223

Baird, Mike, 249-253

bath, 51, 64, 68, 78-9, 86, 89, 129, 150, 160, 171

Beer and Bubs, xv, 77, 255

birth, *see* childbirth

birth attendant, *see* doula

birth ball, 20, 21, 51, 82, 83

Birth Partner, The (Simpkin), 128

birth plan, xiii, 11-13, 129, 147

blood loss, 22, 183

bonding, 1, 3, 9, 31, 196-7, 201, 208, 210, 211, 213

BPA/Bisphenol A, 244-5

Braxton Hicks, 127

breastfeeding: 31, 33, 68, 183, 195, 198-9, 201, 212, 221, 222, 224, 225, 226, 241-7; diet, 243-4, 247; establishing after birth, 195, 198; hardware, 244-5; hydration, 226; nipple trauma, 242-3; problems with, 241-7; professional help, 241-2

Caesarean: 10, 14, 31, 99, 113, 127, 148, 207-13; Australian statistics, 207; elective 207; emergency 53, 113, 128; operating theatre, 210; pain relief, 211-212; rates, 207; risks, 207; theatre attire, 208; unscheduled, 207; fathers in attendance, 208-9; feelings 208

caregivers, conflict with, 114-5, 116

catecholamine, 196

cervical dilation: explanation of, 127; progress, 151; dilation, visual and verbal cues, 170

childbirth horror stories, 10-1, 59, 111

childbirth plan, *see* birth plan

childbirth preferences, 10, 11, 12, 15, 67, 112-13, 114

childbirth support people, 29-37

childbirth: choices *see* childbirth preferences, 134; fear of 3, 4, 13, 19, 31, 59, 61, 69, 85, 184; history of, 1-2; judgements, 10, 43; mobile phone use during, 80, 131, 143, 147, 148, 183, 187; music in, 80, 89, 129, 146; sense of failure, 12, 46, 49, 88, 207; time/timing of, 44, 46, 48, 53, 60, 62, 63, 131,162-3, 169-70; use of language in, 43, 44-45, 46, 53, 80, 150, 173; videos, 6

circumcision, 227

clary sage oil, *see* essential oils

colostrum, 198

conflict, *see* caregivers, conflict with

contraction: pain, *see* pain; pattern, 134-5, talking during, 43-4, timing of, 134-5

Cook, Cath, 32

Dahlen, Hannah, 3, 30, 62, 64, 68, 88, 115, 170, 196

diathermy, 210

dilation, *see* cervical dilation

dog: preparation of, 223

doppler, 147

doula: birth, 5, 12, 19, 20, 29-33, 37, 43, 45, 50, 52, 80, 86, 97, 98, 113, 132, 160, 174, 211; postnatal, 222

due date, estimated, 62, 63, 113, 128, 131

due date, overdue, 63, 128

endorphins, 4, 67-8, 69, 82

epidural: 84-86; application of, 87; avoiding, 84-6; effects, 87, 199; rates, 31; risks, 84-5; sleep during, 149; walking, 87-88

episiotomy, 184, 230

essential oils: clary sage, 79; grapefruit, 81; lime, 81, 83; mandarin, 81; peppermint, 81; sandalwood, 79

family, boundaries, 131, 195-6, 223-4, 211

father, catching baby, 175, 177

father, feelings at moment of birth, 176

fatherhood, *see* parenting

fathers, no desire to be at birth, 3-4

fathers: alcohol, sedation, 47; at birth, 1-6; complaining, 46, 48, 53; personal hygiene, 51

Ferguson, Mark, 179-182

foetal monitor, 87, 147, 148, 161 *see also* doppler

Food Rules (Pollan), 227

food: after the birth, 197-8; during birth, 52, 129

formula feeding, 246-247

Galilee, David, 103-109

Galilee, Michelle, 96-97

gas, *see* nitrous oxide

Gosens, Gerrard, 215-218

grapefruit oil, *see* essential oils

Green, Danny, 91-94

grief, 95, 96, 97-8, 100

Haemorrhagic Disease of the
Newborn, 200
heat, 78, 79, 144
heat packs, 78, 83, 89, 98, 129, 143
Hingston-Jones, Vicky, 79, 80-81, 133
homebirth, 1, 5, 10, 161, 170, 184, 187
Hone, Digby, 119-124
hormones, see adrenalin, endorphins,
oxytocin and relaxin
horror stories, see childbirth, horror
stories
hospital: birth suite set up, 146-7;
night entrance, 145-6; packing
list, 129-30; recovery ward, 113,
211; private, 14, 30, 161, 170, 184;
public, 14, 16, 113, 130, 171, 184;
system, protocol, 113-4, 117, 171,
177, transfer to, 144-5
hydration, 51-2, 134, 135, 143-4, 147,
199, 226, 244, 247
hypnosis, 77

induction: 62; natural techniques,
63-9; nipple stimulation, 64; sex,
63-4, 134; sweeping membranes, 62;
walking, 63
infant child restraint, 130

Keogh, John Dr, 11-12, 15, 32, 34, 59,
66-7, 84, 86-7, 173, 176, 208-9
Khalsa, Akal, 23, 24, 25, 26, 27, 61,
169-70, 243-4, 246

labour: defecating in, 161-3; farting in,
162; first stage, 143-51; induction of,
62-5, 69, 113; second stage, 169-77;
spontaneous, 62, 63, 69; stall, 50,
69, 146, 149-50, 151; transition,
159-63
language, see childbirth, use of
language in
lime oil, see essential oils
Lotus birth, 187
Love, Denise, 12-13, 31-2, 33-4, 35-6,
48, 52, 65-6, 86,

mandarin oil, see essential oils
marriage, status quo after birth, 201
massage oil: 79, 129; coconut oil, 61;
sweet almond oil, 61, 79, 133
mastitis, 241, 245-6, 247
maternal effort, 169, 177, see also
labour, third stage
Maxwell, David, 235-40
meconium, 130, 183
midwives, 13-6, 30-1, 36, 45, 113-16,
147, 169, 170, 171, 196, 198, 211,
see also caregivers, conflict with
mirror, use of during labour, 35, 173
miscarriage, 95-101
modesty, 13
morphine, 67, 84-9, 211-2
mothers at birth, 34-7
music, 80, 89, 129, 146

nappy changes, 224
nappy options/choices, 229
neocortex, 44-5
newborn procedures, 196
nitrous oxide, 83, 86, 89

obstetricians, 13, 14-5, 30, 84, 113, 150, 161, 170, 175, *see also* caregivers, conflict with

Occhilupo, Mark, 165-168

Odent, Michel Dr, 2-3, 197

Osborne, Paul, 55-8

oxytocin, 64, 68, 69, 183, 198, 200

pain management arsenal, 77, 78-89

pain management routine, 82, 89, 143, 145, 147, 149, 151, 160, 163

pain management, movement, 82, 88, 89, 171

pain: back, 84; description of, 60; drugs, 83-9; fear of, 59, natural management of, 77-83; thresholds, 60-1; pharmacological relief, *see* pain, drugs

parenting: 222, 223, 232-3; adjustment to, 226

paternity leave, 128

pelvic floor, 173-4, 177, 228, 231-2

peppermint oil, *see* essential oils

perineal: massage, 61; tearing, 59, 61, 171, 184-5, 212; tearing, positions for prevention, 171-172, 177; tearing, repair, 184-6

Perry, Bruce, 29, 48, 132, 186

Perry, Lucy and Bruce: birth stories, 19-27

Perry, Lucy: qualifications, 4-5

pethidine, 84, 89

placenta: delivery of, 183-4; keeping the, 186-7

Pollan, Michael, 227

Porter, Ric, xi-xiii

position: anterior, 62-6, 69; influence, 64-7; posterior, 64, 66-7, 84

postnatal: bleeding, 96, 129, 200, 228; depression, 225; depression, contributing factors, 225; diet, 226-7; domestic help, 222; exercise, 228, 230; hormones, 221; open house, 224; visitors, 223

pregnancy loss, *see* stillbirth and miscarriage

Pregnancy Loss: Surviving Miscarriage and Stillbirth (Taylor), 95-6

prelabour, 127-135

primal brain, 44-45, 150

pushing, *see* labour, second stage

pushing technique, 172-3

relaxin, 184, 232

rupture of membranes, *see* waters breaking

sandalwood oil, *see* essential oils

Scientification of Love (Odent), 197

sex after birth, 230-2, 233

Sex Diaries, The (Arndt), 231-2

sex during labour, 63-4, 134

shower, 51, 79, 89, 129, 150, 160, 162, 171, 200

Simkins, Penny, 128

sisters at birth, 33, 35-6

skin-to-skin contact, 196-8, 201, 210, 211-2

smell, 51, 79, 80-1, 197, 198, 200, 210, 211

sound, 80, 83, 143, 161, 170
sterile water injections, 84, 89
stillbirth, 95-101
support people, 29-37
sweeping membranes, 62
Sykes, Gary Dr, 14-15
Syntocinon, 31, 114, 149, 183

taste, 82, 197-8
Taylor, Zoe, 95-6
tearing, *see* perineal tearing
Teo, Charlie Dr, 153-8
Tomkins, James, 71-5
touch, 78-9,
transition, *see* labour, transition
Treseder, Paul, 39-42

umbilical cord, 175; around neck, 175;
    blood, 184; cutting of, 184, 187;
    stump, 199-200, 224
urge to push, 161-2, 169-71

vaginal examinations, 148, 150-1, 186
vernix, 199, 201
Vincent, Tim, 189-93
visual focus, 82, 83, 89, 129, 173
vitamin K, 200
vocalisation, 80, 83, 89, 143, 161
vomiting, 81, 83-4, 131, 147

water birth, 171
waters breaking, 95, 130, 131-2

yoga, 228-30, *see also* postnatal
    exercise